Don't Lose Hope

Aaidh

Copyright ©

King Fahd National Library Cataloging-in-Publication Data

All rights reserved. No part of this book may be reproduced or transmitted in any form or by any means, electronic or mechanical, including photocopying, recording, or by any information storage and retrieval system, without written permission from the Publisher.

Whenever you are sad, remember the favors of Allah (God) so that you might succeed. Take a quick look around you right now. He has given you so much: trees, fruits, nuts, birds, oxygen, water, and much more, yet you do not see anything. You have all that life has to offer, yet you remain unhappy. Why?

Whosoever is on the earth and in the heavens asks and begs of Him. Each day God has a matter to bring forth [such as giving honor to some, disgrace to some, life to some, and death to others] (Quran 55:29)

يَسْأَلُهُۥ مَن فِى ٱلسَّمَٰوَٰتِ وَٱلْأَرْضِ ۚ كُلَّ يَوْمٍ هُوَ فِى شَأْنٍ ﴿٢٩﴾

- When the seas and the winds are turbulent, the occupants of the land and sea, cry out only to Him for mercy.

- When the camels are lost in the hot desert, the travelers cry out only to Him for direction and mercy.
- When the earth trembles and rumbles, the afflicted cry out only to Him for mercy.
- When barriers are placed and the doors are shut, they cry out only to Him for mercy.
- When all hope is lost, and there are no exits, they cry out only to Him for mercy.
- When all paths and roads are blocked, causing the soul and the heart to feel constricted and suffocated, they cry out only to Him for mercy.

To Allah alone ascend all that is good: your deeds, words, sincere supplication, the pleas and the tears of the innocent, and the prayers of the afflicted.

Our hands, arms, and eyes are extended to Him for His mercy, to rescues us in times of hardship and misfortune. Our tongues chant His name and glory, and cries out for His help, forgiveness and mercy. Our hearts find peace when He is near. Our souls and eyes find rest, our nerves are soothed, and our minds find peace.

Allah is always very Gracious and Kind to all His creations. Allah gives provisions to whom He wills. And He is the Powerful and the Exalted in Might. (Quran 42:19)

ٱللَّهُ لَطِيفٌۢ بِعِبَادِهِۦ يَرْزُقُ مَن يَشَآءُۖ وَهُوَ ٱلْقَوِىُّ ٱلْعَزِيزُ ﴿١٩﴾

Have you ever seen or known anyone that is similar to Him? He is the One who guides, the One who protects, and the One Who forgives. There is nothing beyond Him or like Him. He is the All-Hearer, the All-Knower, and the All-Seer.

He is the Lord of the heavens, the earth, and whatever is between them, so worship Him and have patience. Do you know of any similarity to Him? (Quran 19:65)

رَبُّ ٱلسَّمَٰوَٰتِ وَٱلۡأَرۡضِ وَمَا بَيۡنَهُمَا فَٱعۡبُدۡهُ وَٱصۡطَبِرۡ لِعِبَٰدَتِهِۦۚ هَلۡ تَعۡلَمُ لَهُۥ سَمِيࣰّا ۝

God: He is the only thought of when utter strength, glory, and wisdom come to mind.

God: He is the only thought of when kindness, care, support, love, and mercy come to mind.

The Day they come forth nothing concerning them will be concealed from Allah. To whom belongs [all] sovereignty this Day? To Allah, the One, the Prevailing. (Quran 40:16)

يَوْمَ هُم بَارِزُونَ ۖ لَا يَخْفَىٰ عَلَى ٱللَّهِ مِنْهُمْ شَىْءٌ ۚ لِّمَنِ ٱلْمُلْكُ ٱلْيَوْمَ ۖ لِلَّهِ ٱلْوَٰحِدِ ٱلْقَهَّارِ ﴿١٦﴾

O'Allah! Let relief take the place of sorrow, make joy come after grief, and let peace take the place of war and fear.

O' Allah: Relieve the tired souls and hearts with the strength of faith. We seek refuge in You from being afraid of anyone but You, from depending upon anyone but in You, from putting our life and trust in anyone but in You, and from worshiping or invoking anyone but You. You are the King of kings, the Supreme, the One and Only.

Be Thankful

God has completed and perfected His Graces upon you. He has given you faith and guided you for doing righteous deeds. He has given you pleasures and delights in this life, and then a better life in the Hereafter in Paradise.

You have at your disposal two eyes to see, two ears to hear, a tongue and lips to taste and to speak, and two hands and two legs to work, to eat, and to live.

Then which of the Blessings of your Lord will you both (jinns and men) deny? (Quran 55:13)

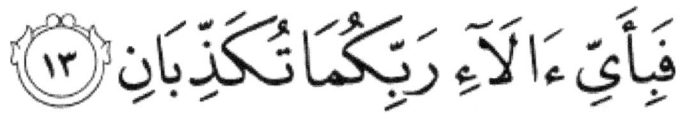

Can you walk without your feet? Should you take it lightly that you sleep soundly while sorrow, hunger, and pain hinders the sleep of so many? Should you forget that you fill your stomach each day with tasty foods and cool water, while the pleasure of any food and clean water is impossible for so many?

Pause for a moment and look at the moon and the stars above you. Say it is He Who has created them for you, and endowed you with hearing (ears), seeing (eyes), and hearts. Little thanks you give. (Quran 67:23)

قُلْ هُوَ ٱلَّذِىٓ أَنشَأَكُمْ وَجَعَلَ لَكُمُ ٱلسَّمْعَ وَٱلْأَبْصَٰرَ وَٱلْأَفْـِٔدَةَ ۖ قَلِيلًا مَّا تَشْكُرُونَ ﴿٢٣﴾

Look at your health and be grateful that you are still alive and have been saved from illness. And when I am sick, then He restores me to health. (Quran 26:80)

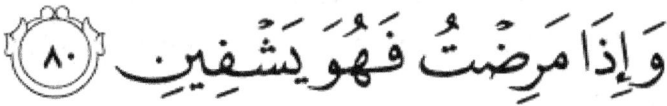

Reflect on your powers of reasoning and remember those that suffer from mental ailments. And when he attained his full strength, We bestowed upon him judgment and knowledge. And thus do We reward the doers of good. (Quran 28:14)

وَلَمَّا بَلَغَ أَشُدَّهُۥ وَٱسْتَوَىٰٓ ءَاتَيْنَٰهُ حُكْمًا وَعِلْمًا وَكَذَٰلِكَ نَجْزِى ٱلْمُحْسِنِينَ ۝

Would you sell your ability to see, smell, and hear for a mountain in gold, or your ability to walk and to speak for a Kingdom of your own? You have been given abundant favors, yet you feign ignorance.

Allah presents an example: a city which was safe and secure, its provision came to it in abundance from all directions, but it denied the favors of Allah. So Allah made it taste the envelopment of hunger and fear for what they had done. (Quran 16:112)

$$\text{وَضَرَبَ ٱللَّهُ مَثَلًا قَرْيَةً كَانَتْ ءَامِنَةً مُّطْمَئِنَّةً يَأْتِيهَا رِزْقُهَا رَغَدًا مِّن كُلِّ مَكَانٍ فَكَفَرَتْ بِأَنْعُمِ ٱللَّهِ فَأَذَاقَهَا ٱللَّهُ لِبَاسَ ٱلْجُوعِ وَٱلْخَوْفِ بِمَا كَانُوا۟ يَصْنَعُونَ ۝}$$

What about the warm bread, the cold milk, the cool water, the good health? Do you remain sad and low? You always dream about what you do not have and are ungrateful for what Allah has given you. You are sad by what is lost, yet you have been given the keys to so many blessings. Contemplate and be thankful.

And if only the people had thanked Allah, We would have opened upon them blessings from the heaven and the earth; but they denied us, so We seized them for what they were doing." (Quran 7:96)

وَلَوْ أَنَّ أَهْلَ ٱلْقُرَىٰٓ ءَامَنُواْ وَٱتَّقَوْاْ لَفَتَحْنَا عَلَيْهِم بَرَكَٰتٍ مِّنَ ٱلسَّمَآءِ وَٱلْأَرْضِ وَلَٰكِن كَذَّبُواْ فَأَخَذْنَٰهُم بِمَا كَانُواْ يَكْسِبُونَ ﴿٩٦﴾

Let go of the past

There are too many good things that surround us every day but we miss them by worrying about the past or being fearful of the future. Shift your thoughts away from what is not working to what is. Say to those who have disbelieved, if they stop, their past will be forgiven. But if they return (thereto), then the examples of those (punished) before them have already preceded (as a warning). (Quran 8:38)

قُل لِّلَّذِينَ كَفَرُوٓاْ إِن يَنتَهُواْ يُغۡفَرۡ لَهُم مَّا قَدۡ سَلَفَ وَإِن يَعُودُواْ فَقَدۡ مَضَتۡ سُنَّتُ ٱلۡأَوَّلِينَ ﴿٣٨﴾

The mistakes of the past are done; they cannot be redone. Sadness and sorrow cannot make things right, and depression will never bring them back to life. The past is something you will never be able to change. The past is non-existent, dead, gone forever.

Do not try to live in the bad dreams, the nightmares, of the past. Rescue yourself from those ghosts. The choice is yours. You are only human. You were born to make mistakes. Simply put, if you have never made a mistake in your life, then that means that you have never taken a risk.

But remember, you cannot turn back time. By residing in the past and its events, you place your wellbeing in danger. It is okay to be sad when you mess up, but do not dwell for too long. The mistakes have already been made, and you cannot erase the fact that they happened. Learn from your mistakes and move on heroically and bravely.

Now is what you have

Worrying about yesterday is about as productive as trying to saw sawdust. Have you ever sawed wood? You saw, the wood gets cut, and then you use the wood for something. Ever sawed sawdust? No? Do you know why? Because there is no point to it!

What purpose would it serve? It would be a colossal waste of time. Worrying about things that have gone is also a colossal waste of time.

It is impossible to go back and change anything that happened yesterday. You must live in the now. The past is gone and the future is yours to make and color. Life is very rough at times. It is always difficult to move on, but please remember that everything on earth marches forward preparing for a new season, and so should you. The enjoyment of this world is very little, but the Hereafter is better for one who fears Allah. Injustice will not be done to you, [even] as much as a thread [inside a date seed]." (Quran 4:77)

قُل مَتَـٰعُ ٱلدُّنْيَا قَلِيلٌ وَٱلْـَٔاخِرَةُ خَيْرٌ لِّمَنِ ٱتَّقَىٰ وَلَا تُظْلَمُونَ فَتِيلًا ﴿٧٧﴾

If you have had a very stressful day, sleep is your medicine. Islam has great interest in sleep. Sleep is considered as one of the signs of the greatness of Allah. Sleep is mentioned frequently in the Quran.

A very well-known verse says: "And of His signs is your sleep by night and day and your seeking of His bounty. Indeed in that are signs for a people who listen." [Quran 30:23].

وَمِنْ ءَايَٰتِهِۦ مَنَامُكُم بِٱلَّيْلِ وَٱلنَّهَارِ وَٱبْتِغَآؤُكُم مِّن فَضْلِهِۦٓ إِنَّ فِى ذَٰلِكَ لَءَايَٰتٍ لِّقَوْمٍ يَسْمَعُونَ ﴿٢٣﴾

The Quran frequently mentions sleep: And it is He who has made the night for you as clothing and sleep [a means for] rest and has made the day a resurrection. (Quran 25:47)

وَهُوَ ٱلَّذِى جَعَلَ لَكُمُ ٱلَّيْلَ لِبَاسًا وَٱلنَّوْمَ سُبَاتًا وَجَعَلَ ٱلنَّهَارَ نُشُورًا ﴿٤٧﴾

And it is He who takes your souls by night and knows what you have committed by day. Then He revives you therein that a specified term may be fulfilled. Then to

Him will be your return; then He will inform you about what you used to do." (Quran 6:60)

$$\text{وَهُوَ ٱلَّذِى يَتَوَفَّىٰكُم بِٱلَّيْلِ وَيَعْلَمُ مَا جَرَحْتُم بِٱلنَّهَارِ ثُمَّ يَبْعَثُكُمْ فِيهِ لِيُقْضَىٰٓ أَجَلٌ مُّسَمًّى ۖ ثُمَّ إِلَيْهِ مَرْجِعُكُمْ ثُمَّ يُنَبِّئُكُم بِمَا كُنتُمْ تَعْمَلُونَ ۝}$$

Mention the story when Joseph said to his father, "O my father, indeed I have seen [in my sleep, a dream] eleven stars and the sun and the moon; I saw them prostrating to me." (Quran 12:4)

$$\text{إِذْ قَالَ يُوسُفُ لِأَبِيهِ يَٰٓأَبَتِ إِنِّى رَأَيْتُ أَحَدَ عَشَرَ كَوْكَبًا وَٱلشَّمْسَ وَٱلْقَمَرَ رَأَيْتُهُمْ لِى سَٰجِدِينَ ۝}$$

Muslims believe that dreams appearing in the last third of the night are more truthful. This correlates with the current scientific understanding that the longest periods of REM sleep occurs during the last third of the nocturnal sleep period, when dream imagination is most active.

He said, "O my son, indeed I have seen in a dream that I [must] sacrifice you, so see what you think." He said, "O my father, do as you are commanded. You will find me, if Allah wills, of the steadfast." (Quran 37:102)

فَلَمَّا بَلَغَ مَعَهُ ٱلسَّعْىَ قَالَ يَٰبُنَىَّ إِنِّىٓ أَرَىٰ فِى ٱلْمَنَامِ أَنِّىٓ أَذْبَحُكَ فَٱنظُرْ مَاذَا تَرَىٰ ۚ قَالَ يَٰٓأَبَتِ ٱفْعَلْ مَا تُؤْمَرُ ۖ سَتَجِدُنِىٓ إِن شَآءَ ٱللَّهُ مِنَ ٱلصَّٰبِرِينَ ۝١٠٢

If you wake up in the morning, do not expect to see the evening.

Live and remember Allah as though this minute is all that you have. Yesterday is gone with its good and evil, but tomorrow has not yet arrived.

Indeed, in the creation of the heavens and earth, and the alternation of the night and the day ... are signs for a people who use reason. (Quran 2:164)

إِنَّ فِى خَلْقِ ٱلسَّمَٰوَٰتِ وَٱلْأَرْضِ وَٱخْتِلَٰفِ ٱلَّيْلِ وَٱلنَّهَارِ وَٱلْفُلْكِ ٱلَّتِى تَجْرِى فِى ٱلْبَحْرِ بِمَا يَنفَعُ ٱلنَّاسَ وَمَا أَنزَلَ ٱللَّهُ مِنَ ٱلسَّمَآءِ مِن مَّآءٍ فَأَحْيَا بِهِ ٱلْأَرْضَ بَعْدَ مَوْتِهَا وَبَثَّ فِيهَا مِن كُلِّ دَآبَّةٍ وَتَصْرِيفِ ٱلرِّيَٰحِ وَٱلسَّحَابِ ٱلْمُسَخَّرِ بَيْنَ ٱلسَّمَآءِ وَٱلْأَرْضِ لَءَايَٰتٍ لِّقَوْمٍ يَعْقِلُونَ ۝١٦٤

Your life's span is but one night, as if you were born at the beginning of it, and you are gone at the end of it.

With this attitude, you will not be fixated over the past, with all its fears, and the worries of tomorrow, with all its uncertainties. So live for that night. Remember Allah with much remembrance and glorify Him, and pray with a wakeful heart.

Indeed, for the believing men and believing women, the obedient men and obedient women, the truthful men and truthful women, the patient men and patient women, the humble men and humble women, the charitable men and charitable women, the fasting men and fasting women, the men who guard their private parts and the women who do so, and the men who remember Allah often and the women who do so - for them Allah has prepared forgiveness and a beautiful reward. (Quran 33:35)

إِنَّ ٱلْمُسْلِمِينَ وَٱلْمُسْلِمَٰتِ وَٱلْمُؤْمِنِينَ وَٱلْمُؤْمِنَٰتِ وَٱلْقَٰنِتِينَ وَٱلْقَٰنِتَٰتِ وَٱلصَّٰدِقِينَ وَٱلصَّٰدِقَٰتِ وَٱلصَّٰبِرِينَ وَٱلصَّٰبِرَٰتِ وَٱلْخَٰشِعِينَ وَٱلْخَٰشِعَٰتِ وَٱلْمُتَصَدِّقِينَ وَٱلْمُتَصَدِّقَٰتِ وَٱلصَّٰٓئِمِينَ وَٱلصَّٰٓئِمَٰتِ وَٱلْحَٰفِظِينَ فُرُوجَهُمْ وَٱلْحَٰفِظَٰتِ وَٱلذَّٰكِرِينَ ٱللَّهَ كَثِيرًا وَٱلذَّٰكِرَٰتِ أَعَدَّ ٱللَّهُ لَهُم مَّغْفِرَةً وَأَجْرًا عَظِيمًا ۝

Recite God's Book and remember Allah with much sincerity. In each day you must be balanced in all your affairs, satisfied with your allotted share, and concerned with your health and appearance.

(Allah) said: "So hold that which I have given you and be of the grateful." (Quran 7:144). And eat of the lawful things that We have provided you with, and be grateful. (Quran 2:172)

قَالَ يَٰمُوسَىٰٓ إِنِّى ٱصْطَفَيْتُكَ عَلَى ٱلنَّاسِ بِرِسَٰلَٰتِى وَبِكَلَٰمِى فَخُذْ مَآ ءَاتَيْتُكَ وَكُن مِّنَ ٱلشَّٰكِرِينَ ﴿١٤٤﴾

يَٰٓأَيُّهَا ٱلَّذِينَ ءَامَنُوا۟ كُلُوا۟ مِن طَيِّبَٰتِ مَا رَزَقْنَٰكُمْ وَٱشْكُرُوا۟ لِلَّهِ إِن كُنتُمْ إِيَّاهُ تَعْبُدُونَ ﴿١٧٢﴾

Who rescues you from the darkness of the land and the sea, when you call upon Him in humility and in secret (saying): If He (Allah) only saves us from this (danger), we shall truly be grateful. (Quran 6:63)

قُلْ مَن يُنَجِّيكُم مِّن ظُلُمَٰتِ ٱلْبَرِّ وَٱلْبَحْرِ تَدْعُونَهُۥ تَضَرُّعًا وَخُفْيَةً لَّئِنْ أَنجَىٰنَا مِنْ هَٰذِهِۦ لَنَكُونَنَّ مِنَ ٱلشَّٰكِرِينَ ﴿٦٣﴾

It is He who subjected the sea for you to eat from it tender meat and to extract from it ornaments which you wear. And you see the ships plowing through it, and [He subjected it] that you may seek of His bounty; and perhaps you will be grateful. (Quran 16:14)

وَهُوَ ٱلَّذِى سَخَّرَ ٱلْبَحْرَ لِتَأْكُلُوا۟ مِنْهُ لَحْمًا طَرِيًّا وَتَسْتَخْرِجُوا۟ مِنْهُ حِلْيَةً تَلْبَسُونَهَا وَتَرَى ٱلْفُلْكَ مَوَاخِرَ فِيهِ وَلِتَبْتَغُوا۟ مِن فَضْلِهِۦ وَلَعَلَّكُمْ تَشْكُرُونَ ﴿١٤﴾

<u>Free your heart from hatred and anger</u>

Engrave this into your heart: Today might be your last. So enjoy today and forget about yesterday. If you have eaten warm, fresh pancakes today, then what do yesterday's dry bread, and tomorrow's anticipated bread matter? No blame will there be upon you today.

Allah will forgive you; and He is the most forgiving and compassionate. (Quran 12:92)

$$\text{قَالَ لَا تَثْرِيبَ عَلَيْكُمُ ٱلْيَوْمَ يَغْفِرُ ٱللَّهُ لَكُمْ وَهُوَ أَرْحَمُ ٱلرَّاحِمِينَ ﴿٩٢﴾}$$

If you truthfully believe that today is your last day to live, you will enjoy every second of your day. Talk to everyone that you meet. Expand your interests, build your confidence, and purify your actions and deeds. Refine your speech and utter neither evil nor obscene speech. And do not backbite anyone. The Messenger of Allah (peace be upon him) said: "Do not backbite each other, and do not search for the faults of others, for if anyone searches for their faults, Allah will search for your faults, and if Allah searches for the fault of anyone, He disgraces them in His House."

"O you who have believed, avoid much [negative] assumption. Indeed, some assumption is sin. And do not spy or backbite each other. Would one of you like to eat the flesh of his brother when dead? You would detest it. And fear Allah; indeed, Allah is Accepting of repentance and Merciful." (Quran 49:12)

يَٰٓأَيُّهَا ٱلَّذِينَ ءَامَنُوا۟ ٱجْتَنِبُوا۟ كَثِيرًا مِّنَ ٱلظَّنِّ إِنَّ بَعْضَ ٱلظَّنِّ إِثْمٌ ۖ وَلَا تَجَسَّسُوا۟ وَلَا يَغْتَب بَّعْضُكُم بَعْضًا ۚ أَيُحِبُّ أَحَدُكُمْ أَن يَأْكُلَ لَحْمَ أَخِيهِ مَيْتًا فَكَرِهْتُمُوهُ ۚ وَٱتَّقُوا۟ ٱللَّهَ ۚ إِنَّ ٱللَّهَ تَوَّابٌ رَّحِيمٌ ﴿١٢﴾

So today strive to be obedient to your Lord, pray in the best way that you can. Do more voluntary acts of worship, such extra prayers and fasting. Recite God's Book, and read beneficial books. Try planting goodness into your heart, and you will reap friends.

If you plant honesty, you will reap trust.

If you plant humility, you will reap greatness.

If you plant perseverance, you will reap victory.

If you plant consideration, you will reap harmony.

If you plant hard work, you will reap success.

If you plant forgiveness, you will reap happiness.

If you plant faith, you will reap miracles.

If you plant dishonesty, you will reap distrust.

If you plant selfishness, you will reap loneliness.

If you plant pride, you will reap destruction.

If you plant envy, you will reap trouble.

If you plant laziness, you will reap stagnation.

If you plant bitterness, you will reap isolation.

If you plant greed, you will reap loss.

If you plant gossip, you will reap enemies.

If you plant worries, you will reap wrinkles.

If you plant sin, you will reap guilt.

You reap what you sow. The seeds that you scatter today will make life worse or better for you. Focus to become a better you. Believe in yourself or no one else will. So focus your time and efforts and you can become the best version of yourself. Take risks that makes you happy, and push forward regardless of the odds and obstacles. And never ask yourself what the world needs; ask yourself what makes you happy, what makes you come alive, then go do that. Because what the world needs is people who have come alive.

Never worry about money. Allah will never let you down. Waste your money and you are only out of money, but waste your time and you have lost a part of your life. Never be afraid of failing. Look at failure as proof that you are doing something. Accept failure, but never accept not trying. So if you have a dream of doing something, do it. If people are not laughing at your dream, then your dream is not big enough.

Volunteering is one of the most rewarding things that you can do. Visit the sick, guide someone who is lost, and help to feed the hungry. Lift up the weak and enable them to stand up on their own two feet. Stand side by side with the oppressed and the weak. Respect your parents and teachers. Be very merciful and compassionate to the young and to all of Allah's creatures, and be reverent to the old.

Forget about yesterday and tomorrow! Focus on today!

Our lives have meaning, and our actions have vast implications on the well-being our family and this beautiful planet. Some days you wake up in the morning, look out at the day, blue sky, fluffy clouds, then go outside and ten minutes later you have lost the will to live. As we go through our lives we take on the expanding burden of our own distress, as we are abandoned, broken apart, betrayed, isolated, lost and hurt. This is essentially part of what it is to be alive. This despair will overwhelm us and turn inward into bitterness, resentment and hatred, worse, we will take it out upon the ones closest to us if we do not actively live our lives in the service of others and use what power we have to reduce each other's suffering.

This is the key to living. This is the remedy to our own suffering; our own feelings of separateness and of disconnectedness. And it is the essential antidote our loneliness. So do not weaken and do not grieve, and you will be superior if you are [true] believers. (Quran, 3:139)

وَلَا تَهِنُوا۟ وَلَا تَحْزَنُوا۟ وَأَنتُمُ ٱلْأَعْلَوْنَ إِن كُنتُم مُّؤْمِنِينَ ﴿١٣٩﴾

Do not cry over yesterday's spilled milk or about the lost dreams of yesteryear. Say you will never see me thinking about you, not even for a moment, because you have departed and gone away from me never to return. Yesterday is now history and tomorrow is a mystery in the realm of the unseen. So say I will not be preoccupied by thoughts of you.

I will not be day-dreaming about what is to come, because you are nothing until I create you. Today is your day. And the Events ordained by Allah will come to pass, so do not seek to hasten them. (Quran 16:1)

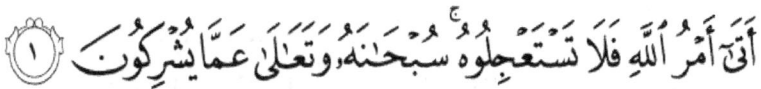

Do not think about and rush things that have yet to happen. It is not very wise to pick fruits before they ripen. Likewise, tomorrow is non-existent. It has no life today. So do not exhaust yourself thinking about things that cause anxiety and fear. Why should you worry about future events if you have no control over them? Why should you be occupied by their thoughts, especially when you do not even know if you will be alive? Let tomorrow be a mystery. You have nothing to fear as long it is today.

Tomorrow is a bridge that you will not cross until you reach it. Who knows, perhaps the bridge will collapse before you arrive, or you may actually reach it and cross without harm.

"Never say about anything, 'Indeed, I will do that tomorrow,' Except [when adding], 'If Allah wills.'" (Quran 18:23)

وَلَا تَقُولَنَّ لِشَايْءٍ إِنِّي فَاعِلٌ ذَٰلِكَ غَدًا ﴿٢٣﴾

Only Allah [alone] has knowledge of tomorrow. He sends down the rain and knows what is in the wombs. And no soul perceives what it will earn tomorrow, and no soul perceives in what land it will die. Indeed, Allah is Knowing of everything. (Quran 31:34)

إِنَّ ٱللَّهَ عِندَهُۥ عِلْمُ ٱلسَّاعَةِ وَيُنَزِّلُ ٱلْغَيْثَ وَيَعْلَمُ مَا فِى ٱلْأَرْحَامِ ۖ وَمَا تَدْرِى نَفْسٌ مَّاذَا تَكْسِبُ غَدًا ۖ وَمَا تَدْرِى نَفْسٌۢ بِأَىِّ أَرْضٍ تَمُوتُ ۚ إِنَّ ٱللَّهَ عَلِيمٌ خَبِيرٌۢ ﴿٣٤﴾

O you who have believed, fear Allah. And let every soul look to what it has put forth for tomorrow - and fear Allah. Indeed, Allah is acquainted with what you do. (Quran 59:18)

يَـٰٓأَيُّهَا ٱلَّذِينَ ءَامَنُوا۟ ٱتَّقُوا۟ ٱللَّهَ وَلْتَنظُرْ نَفْسٌ مَّا قَدَّمَتْ لِغَدٍ ۖ وَٱتَّقُوا۟ ٱللَّهَ ۚ إِنَّ ٱللَّهَ خَبِيرٌۢ بِمَا تَعْمَلُونَ ﴿١٨﴾

To be preoccupied in expectations about the future is looked down upon by Allah since it shows that we have attachment to this earthly life, an attachment that the good believer should reject.

Many people are very fearful of poverty, homelessness, hunger, illness, and disasters. Such fears are inspired by the Devil himself. Satan threatens you with poverty and pushes you to immorality, while Allah promises you forgiveness from Him and bounty. And Allah is all-Encompassing and Knowing. (Quran 2:268)

ٱلشَّيْطَٰنُ يَعِدُكُمُ ٱلْفَقْرَ وَيَأْمُرُكُم بِٱلْفَحْشَآءِ ۖ وَٱللَّهُ يَعِدُكُم مَّغْفِرَةً مِّنْهُ وَفَضْلًا ۗ وَٱللَّهُ وَٰسِعٌ عَلِيمٌ ﴿٢٦٨﴾

His [devil] companion will say, "Our Lord, I did not make him transgress, but he [himself] was in extreme error." (Quran 50:27)

۞ قَالَ قَرِينُهُۥ رَبَّنَا مَآ أَطْغَيْتُهُۥ وَلَٰكِن كَانَ فِى ضَلَٰلٍۭ بَعِيدٍ ﴿٢٧﴾

That is Satan who frightens [you] of his supporters. So fear them not, but fear Me, if you are indeed believers. (Quran 3:175)

إِنَّمَا ذَٰلِكُمُ ٱلشَّيْطَٰنُ يُخَوِّفُ أَوْلِيَآءَهُۥ فَلَا تَخَافُوهُمْ وَخَافُونِ إِن كُنتُم مُّؤْمِنِينَ ﴿١٧٥﴾

The hypocrites are like the example of Satan when he says to man, "I am your friend, Disbelieve in Allah!" But when man disbelieves, he says, "Indeed, I am disassociated from you. Indeed, I fear Allah, Lord of the worlds. (Quran 59:16)

كَمَثَلِ ٱلشَّيْطَٰنِ إِذْ قَالَ لِلْإِنسَٰنِ ٱكْفُرْ فَلَمَّا كَفَرَ قَالَ إِنِّي بَرِيٓءٌ مِّنكَ إِنِّيٓ أَخَافُ ٱللَّهَ رَبَّ ٱلْعَٰلَمِينَ ﴿١٦﴾

He only orders you to evil and immorality and to say about Allah what you do not know. (Quran 2:169)

إِنَّمَا يَأْمُرُكُم بِٱلسُّوٓءِ وَٱلْفَحْشَآءِ وَأَن تَقُولُوا۟ عَلَى ٱللَّهِ مَا لَا تَعْلَمُونَ ﴿١٦٩﴾

Many that disbelieve are those who see themselves starving tomorrow, falling ill, or fearful that the world is about to end. Someone who has no hint as to when they will die, which is everyone, must never busy themselves with such thoughts. Since you are so engaged in the tough toils of today, forget about tomorrow until it is here.

How to deal with ignorance?

Those who are ignorant have even hurled curses at Allah, the Mighty Creator of all that exists, so do not despair of what they have done. And even if We had sent down to them the angels with the message, and the dead stood up and spoke to them of it, and We gathered together every created thing in front of them, they would not believe unless Allah should will. But most of them are ignorant. (Quran 6:111)

﴿ وَلَوْ أَنَّنَا نَزَّلْنَا إِلَيْهِمُ ٱلْمَلَٰٓئِكَةَ وَكَلَّمَهُمُ ٱلْمَوْتَىٰ وَحَشَرْنَا عَلَيْهِمْ كُلَّ شَىْءٍ قُبُلًا مَّا كَانُوا۟ لِيُؤْمِنُوٓا۟ إِلَّآ أَن يَشَآءَ ٱللَّهُ وَلَٰكِنَّ أَكْثَرَهُمْ يَجْهَلُونَ ﴾ (١١١)

You will always have to deal with critics. Criticism is inevitable, and it never ends. But do not despair and serve your Lord till the inevitable come to you. (Quran 15:99)

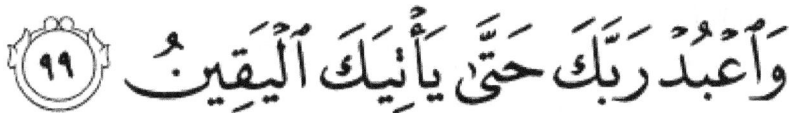

As long as you shine bright, care, give, produce, and others seek you out for your compassionate nature, then condemnation and disapproval will be your lot in life. Unless you can escape from life, they will not stop from censuring you, and from finding faults in your character.

As long as you are a resident of this earth, expect to be wounded, to be in pain, to be criticized, and to be insulted. O you who have believed, let not a people ridicule [another] people; perhaps they may be better than them; nor let women ridicule [other] women; perhaps they may be better than them. And do not insult one another and do not call each other by [offensive] nicknames. Wretched is the name of disobedience after [one's] faith. And whoever does not repent - then it is those who are the wrongdoers. (Quran 49:11)

يَٰٓأَيُّهَا ٱلَّذِينَ ءَامَنُوا۟ لَا يَسْخَرْ قَوْمٌ مِّن قَوْمٍ عَسَىٰٓ أَن يَكُونُوا۟ خَيْرًا مِّنْهُمْ وَلَا نِسَآءٌ مِّن نِّسَآءٍ عَسَىٰٓ أَن يَكُنَّ خَيْرًا مِّنْهُنَّ وَلَا تَلْمِزُوٓا۟ أَنفُسَكُمْ وَلَا تَنَابَزُوا۟ بِٱلْأَلْقَٰبِ بِئْسَ ٱلِٱسْمُ ٱلْفُسُوقُ بَعْدَ ٱلْإِيمَٰنِ وَمَن لَّمْ يَتُبْ فَأُو۟لَٰٓئِكَ هُمُ ٱلظَّٰلِمُونَ ﴿١١﴾

Here is something that you should contemplate: a person laying on the ground does not fall down, and sane people do not kick a rock. So since you shine so brightly, their anger and hate towards you can be attributed to you surpassing them in righteousness, virtue, honesty, manners, knowledge, or wealth.

On the Day you see the believing men and believing women, their shining light proceeding before them and on their right, it will be said:

"Your good tidings today are of gardens beneath which rivers flow, wherein you will abide eternally." That is what the great attainment is. (Quran 57:12)

يَوْمَ تَرَى ٱلْمُؤْمِنِينَ وَٱلْمُؤْمِنَٰتِ يَسْعَىٰ نُورُهُم بَيْنَ أَيْدِيهِمْ وَبِأَيْمَٰنِهِم بُشْرَىٰكُمُ ٱلْيَوْمَ جَنَّٰتٌ تَجْرِى مِن تَحْتِهَا ٱلْأَنْهَٰرُ خَٰلِدِينَ فِيهَا ۚ ذَٰلِكَ هُوَ ٱلْفَوْزُ ٱلْعَظِيمُ ﴿١٢﴾

And some faces that Day shall be Nadirah (shining and so radiant). (Quran 75:22)

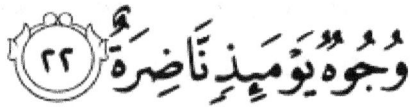

As long as you shine, they will attack you. In their diseased minds they had committed no crimes.

In their eyes you are the transgressor, the wrongdoer, whose wrongs can never be forgiven or corrected. You cannot win unless you abandon your beliefs, and strip yourself of all commendable qualities, so that you become worthless, foolish, and to them, harmless. No matter what you say, they would not hear you, and even if they did, they would not care.

And indeed, every time I invited them that You may forgive them, they put their fingers in their ears, covered themselves with their garments, persisted, and were arrogant with [great] arrogance. (Quran 71:7)

وَإِنِّى كُلَّمَا دَعَوْتُهُمْ لِتَغْفِرَ لَهُمْ جَعَلُوٓا۟ أَصَٰبِعَهُمْ فِىٓ ءَاذَانِهِمْ وَٱسْتَغْشَوْا۟ ثِيَابَهُمْ وَأَصَرُّوا۟ وَٱسْتَكْبَرُوا۟ ٱسْتِكْبَارًا ۝

They want you to turn away from Allah's path. This is exactly what they want you to do. So be very firm and patient when facing their insults and criticism. Tell them this is the path of my Lord. But if you are wounded by their actions and words and let them have influence over you, you will then have fulfilled their desires for them. Instead, remain very patient and continue your good deeds, and forgive them by presenting the kindest manners. Turn away from them and do not feel bothered by their plots. Those are the ones of whom Allah knows what is in their hearts, so turn away from them but admonish them and say to them a far-reaching word. (Quran 4:63)

أُو۟لَٰٓئِكَ ٱلَّذِينَ يَعْلَمُ ٱللَّهُ مَا فِى قُلُوبِهِمْ فَأَعْرِضْ عَنْهُمْ وَعِظْهُمْ وَقُل لَّهُمْ فِىٓ أَنفُسِهِمْ قَوْلًۢا بَلِيغًا ﴿٦٣﴾

Your god is one God. But those who do not believe in the Hereafter - their hearts are disapproving, and they are arrogant. (Quran 16:22)

إِلَٰهُكُمْ إِلَٰهٌ وَٰحِدٌ ۚ فَٱلَّذِينَ لَا يُؤْمِنُونَ بِٱلْءَاخِرَةِ قُلُوبُهُم مُّنكِرَةٌ وَهُم مُّسْتَكْبِرُونَ ﴿٢٢﴾

And when Our verses are recited to them as clear evidences, you recognize in the faces of those who disbelieve disapproval. They are almost on the verge of assaulting those who recite to them Our verses. Say, "Then shall I inform you of [what is] worse than that? [It is] the Fire which Allah has promised those who disbelieve, and wretched is the destination." (Quran 22:72)

Their disapproval of you will only increases you in worth and merit. Verily, you will not be able to silence them but you will be able to bury their criticisms by turning away from them. Say: 'Perish in your rage'. (Quran 3:119)

وَإِذَا تُتْلَىٰ عَلَيْهِمْ ءَايَٰتُنَا بَيِّنَٰتٍ تَعْرِفُ فِى وُجُوهِ ٱلَّذِينَ كَفَرُوا۟ ٱلْمُنكَرَ ۖ يَكَادُونَ يَسْطُونَ بِٱلَّذِينَ يَتْلُونَ عَلَيْهِمْ ءَايَٰتِنَا ۗ قُلْ أَفَأُنَبِّئُكُم بِشَرٍّ مِّن ذَٰلِكُمُ ٱلنَّارُ وَعَدَهَا ٱللَّهُ ٱلَّذِينَ كَفَرُوا۟ ۖ وَبِئْسَ ٱلْمَصِيرُ ﴿٧٢﴾

Never be afraid of them. You will always be able to meet them in their rage and fury by increasing your merits and developing your awareness and talents. If you hope to be loved and accepted by everyone, then you desire the impossible.

Lessons on Gratitude

He showed his gratitude for the favors of Allah, who chose him, and guided him to a Straight Way. (Quran 16:212)

شَاكِرًا لِأَنْعُمِهِ ٱجْتَبَىٰهُ وَهَدَىٰهُ إِلَىٰ صِرَٰطٍ مُّسْتَقِيمٍ ﴿١٢١﴾

Allah, the Almighty, the Creator, the Inventor, the Fashioner, created His servants so that they may worship Him. He has made the earth your couch, and the heavens your canopy; and sent down rain from the heavens; and brought forth therewith Fruits for your sustenance; then set not up rivals unto Allah when ye know (the truth). (Quran 2:22)

ٱلَّذِى جَعَلَ لَكُمُ ٱلْأَرْضَ فِرَٰشًا وَٱلسَّمَآءَ بِنَآءً وَأَنزَلَ مِنَ ٱلسَّمَآءِ مَآءً فَأَخْرَجَ بِهِۦ مِنَ ٱلثَّمَرَٰتِ رِزْقًا لَّكُمْ ۖ فَلَا تَجْعَلُوا۟ لِلَّهِ أَندَادًا وَأَنتُمْ تَعْلَمُونَ ﴿٢٢﴾

Allah provided sustenance for you so that you may be grateful. But many worship others than Him and they are thankful not to Him, but to them. He said: "Do you worship that which you yourselves carve?" (Quran 37:95)

قَالَ أَتَعْبُدُونَ مَا تَنْحِتُونَ ﴿٩٥﴾

Remember Me, I will remember you, and do not be ungrateful. (Quran 2:152)

فَاذْكُرُونِي أَذْكُرْكُمْ وَاشْكُرُوا لِي وَلَا تَكْفُرُونِ ﴿١٥٢﴾

Do not be depressed when you find them ungrateful forgetting your kindness. Many will even look down on you, and see you as their enemy just for showing them kindness. And they could not find any cause at all to bear a grudge, except that Allah and His Messenger had enriched them of His Bounty. (Quran 9:74)

يَحْلِفُونَ بِٱللَّهِ مَا قَالُوا۟ وَلَقَدْ قَالُوا۟ كَلِمَةَ ٱلْكُفْرِ وَكَفَرُوا۟ بَعْدَ إِسْلَـٰمِهِمْ وَهَمُّوا۟ بِمَا لَمْ يَنَالُوا۟ وَمَا نَقَمُوٓا۟ إِلَّآ أَنْ أَغْنَىٰهُمُ ٱللَّهُ وَرَسُولُهُۥ مِن فَضْلِهِۦ ۚ فَإِن يَتُوبُوا۟ يَكُ خَيْرًا لَّهُمْ ۖ وَإِن يَتَوَلَّوْا۟ يُعَذِّبْهُمُ ٱللَّهُ عَذَابًا أَلِيمًا فِى ٱلدُّنْيَا وَٱلْـَٔاخِرَةِ ۚ وَمَا لَهُمْ فِى ٱلْأَرْضِ مِن وَلِىٍّ وَلَا نَصِيرٍ ۝٧٤

Never be sad if you are requited with ingratitude for kindness that you have done. From among the ever-repeating stories of history is the story of Prophet Noah (peace be upon him) and his son. Noah loved his son, he fed him, clothed him and taught him about Allah. Noah stayed up the nights when his son was ill so that his son could sleep. Noah stayed hungry so that his son could eat, and he would work so that his son could feel happiness and comfort. And when Noah's son became older, he rewarded Noah with disobedience, contempt, and disrespect.

And the ship sailed with them through waves like mountains, and Noah called to his son who was apart [from them], "My son, come aboard with us and be not with the disbelievers." (Quran 11:42)

وَهِىَ تَجْرِى بِهِمْ فِى مَوْجٍ كَٱلْجِبَالِ وَنَادَىٰ نُوحٌ ٱبْنَهُۥ وَكَانَ فِى مَعْزِلٍ يَٰبُنَىَّ ٱرْكَب مَّعَنَا وَلَا تَكُن مَّعَ ٱلْكَٰفِرِينَ ﴿٤٢﴾

But he was one of the ungrateful. He said: "I will take refuge on a mountain to protect me from the water." [Noah] said, "There is no protector today from the decree of Allah, except for whom He gives mercy." And the waves came between them, and he was among the drowned. (Quran 11:43)

قَالَ سَـَٔاوِىٓ إِلَىٰ جَبَلٍ يَعْصِمُنِى مِنَ ٱلْمَآءِ قَالَ لَا عَاصِمَ ٱلْيَوْمَ مِنْ أَمْرِ ٱللَّهِ إِلَّا مَن رَّحِمَ وَحَالَ بَيْنَهُمَا ٱلْمَوْجُ فَكَانَ مِنَ ٱلْمُغْرَقِينَ ﴿٤٣﴾

So do not be sad if you are requited with ingratitude for the kindness that you have done. Rejoice for you will be rewarded from Allah for he has unlimited treasures. If you love Allah and His Messenger and the home of the Hereafter - then indeed, Allah has prepared for the doers of good among you a great reward. (Quran 30:29)

$$\text{وَإِن كُنتُنَّ تُرِدْنَ ٱللَّهَ وَرَسُولَهُ وَٱلدَّارَ ٱلْآخِرَةَ فَإِنَّ ٱللَّهَ أَعَدَّ لِلْمُحْسِنَاتِ مِنكُنَّ أَجْرًا عَظِيمًا ﴿٢٩﴾}$$

This is not to say that you should stop doing acts of kindness. But try to be prepared for ingratitude. Do acts of charity only for Allah's pleasure. With such an attitude you will certainly be successful always. The unappreciative person cannot harm you. So praise Allah that you are the obedient servant, and that person is the transgressor, the wrongdoer.

O you who have believed, give from the good things and from that which We have produced for you from the earth. And do not aim toward the defective therefrom, spending [from that] while you would not take it [yourself] except with closed eyes. And know that Allah is Free of need and Praiseworthy. (Quran 2:267)

$$\text{يَٰٓأَيُّهَا ٱلَّذِينَ ءَامَنُوٓاْ أَنفِقُواْ مِن طَيِّبَٰتِ مَا كَسَبْتُمْ وَمِمَّآ أَخْرَجْنَا لَكُم مِّنَ ٱلْأَرْضِ ۖ وَلَا تَيَمَّمُواْ ٱلْخَبِيثَ مِنْهُ تُنفِقُونَ وَلَسْتُم بِـَٔاخِذِيهِ إِلَّآ أَن تُغْمِضُواْ فِيهِ ۚ وَٱعْلَمُوٓاْ أَنَّ ٱللَّهَ غَنِيٌّ حَمِيدٌ ﴿٢٦٧﴾}$$

Always remember that the hand that gives is much better than the hand that receives. Many people are surprised at ingratitude in others. Have they never read this verse and others like it?

And when affliction touches man, he calls upon Us, whether lying on his side or sitting or standing; but when We remove from him his affliction, he continues [in disobedience] as if he had never called upon Us to [remove] an affliction that touched him. (Quran 10:12)

وَإِذَا مَسَّ ٱلْإِنسَٰنَ ٱلضُّرُّ دَعَانَا لِجَنۢبِهِۦ أَوْ قَاعِدًا أَوْ قَآئِمًا فَلَمَّا كَشَفْنَا عَنْهُ ضُرَّهُۥ مَرَّ كَأَن لَّمْ يَدْعُنَآ إِلَىٰ ضُرٍّ مَّسَّهُۥ ۚ كَذَٰلِكَ زُيِّنَ لِلْمُسْرِفِينَ مَا كَانُوا۟ يَعْمَلُونَ ﴿١٢﴾

They say that the pen is mightier than the sword. So do not be sad if you give someone a pen as a gift and he uses it to mock you with it, or if you buy someone a walking cane to help them walk and instead they hit you with it. As I stated earlier, most of us are ungrateful to God, so what thanks should you and I expect?

And remember We said: "Enter this town, and eat of the plenty therein as ye wish; but enter the gate with humility, in posture and in words, and We shall forgive you your faults and increase (the portion of) those who do good." (Quran 2:58)

وَإِذْ قُلْنَا ٱدْخُلُوا۟ هَٰذِهِ ٱلْقَرْيَةَ فَكُلُوا۟ مِنْهَا حَيْثُ شِئْتُمْ رَغَدًا وَٱدْخُلُوا۟ ٱلْبَابَ سُجَّدًا وَقُولُوا۟ حِطَّةٌ نَّغْفِرْ لَكُمْ خَطَٰيَٰكُمْ ۚ وَسَنَزِيدُ ٱلْمُحْسِنِينَ ۝

Verily! Those who believe and those who are Jews and Christians, and Sabians, whoever believes in Allah and the Last Day and do righteous good deeds shall have their reward with their Lord, on them shall be no fear, nor shall they grieve. (Quran 2:62)

إِنَّ ٱلَّذِينَ ءَامَنُوا۟ وَٱلَّذِينَ هَادُوا۟ وَٱلنَّصَٰرَىٰ وَٱلصَّٰبِـِٔينَ مَنْ ءَامَنَ بِٱللَّهِ وَٱلْيَوْمِ ٱلْءَاخِرِ وَعَمِلَ صَٰلِحًا فَلَهُمْ أَجْرُهُمْ عِندَ رَبِّهِمْ وَلَا خَوْفٌ عَلَيْهِمْ وَلَا هُمْ يَحْزَنُونَ ﴿٦٢﴾

And those who believe (in the Oneness of Allah - Islamic Monotheism) and do righteous good deeds, they are dwellers of Paradise, they will dwell therein forever. (Quran 2:82)

وَٱلَّذِينَ ءَامَنُوا۟ وَعَمِلُوا۟ ٱلصَّٰلِحَٰتِ أُو۟لَٰٓئِكَ أَصْحَٰبُ ٱلْجَنَّةِ هُمْ فِيهَا خَٰلِدُونَ ﴿٨٢﴾

And establish prayer and give Zakah, and whatever good you put forward for yourselves - you will find it with Allah. Indeed, Allah of what you do, is Seeing. (Quran 2:110)

وَأَقِيمُوا۟ ٱلصَّلَوٰةَ وَءَاتُوا۟ ٱلزَّكَوٰةَ وَمَا تُقَدِّمُوا۟ لِأَنفُسِكُم مِّنْ خَيْرٍ تَجِدُوهُ عِندَ ٱللَّهِ إِنَّ ٱللَّهَ بِمَا تَعْمَلُونَ بَصِيرٌ ﴿١١٠﴾

Doing Good Deeds Gives Allah's Pleasure

The Messenger of Allah (peace be upon him) taught people to be constructive, beneficial members of their societies; always helping those who are deprived and destitute to the best of their abilities. Every good deed is described as an act of charity, as the Prophet said: "Every person must give charity." They said, "O Messenger of Allah, what if he cannot do that?" He said: "Then let him help one who is in desperate need or do good, and refrain from doing evil, and that will be an act of charity on his part."

And be steadfast in prayer; practice regular charity; and bow down your heads with those who bow down (in worship). (Quran 2:43)

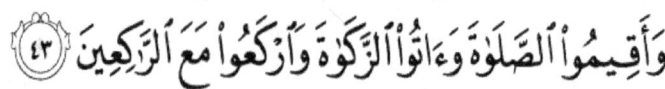

The Messenger of Allah (peace be upon him) said that the first person who benefits from an act of kindness is the giver himself. With time, he will see changes in himself and in his manners. He will find peace and happiness when he sees a smile form on the face of another person. If you ever find yourself in distress or in difficulty situation, show kindness to others, and I promise you that you will find relief and comfort too.

I often had very little money and food, but if I still gave someone something, Allah gave me back ten times what I gave by the end of that day. So always give something, defend and protect the oppressed, help those in pain, be kind to your family, and visit your parents and the sick. If you do all that, you will find happiness from all directions. Do not worship but Allah; and to your parents do good and to the relatives, orphans, and the needy. And speak to people good [words] and establish prayer and give Zakah. (Quran 2:83)

وَإِذْ أَخَذْنَا مِيثَٰقَ بَنِىٓ إِسْرَٰٓءِيلَ لَا تَعْبُدُونَ إِلَّا ٱللَّهَ وَبِٱلْوَٰلِدَيْنِ إِحْسَانًا وَذِى ٱلْقُرْبَىٰ وَٱلْيَتَٰمَىٰ وَٱلْمَسَٰكِينِ وَقُولُوا۟ لِلنَّاسِ حُسْنًا وَأَقِيمُوا۟ ٱلصَّلَوٰةَ وَءَاتُوا۟ ٱلزَّكَوٰةَ ثُمَّ تَوَلَّيْتُمْ إِلَّا قَلِيلًا مِّنكُمْ وَأَنتُم مُّعْرِضُونَ ﴿٨٣﴾

They ask you, [O Muhammad], what they should spend. Say, "Whatever you spend of good is [to be] for parents and relatives and orphans and the needy and the traveler. And whatever you do of good - indeed, Allah is Knowing of it." (Quran 2:15)

يَسْـَٔلُونَكَ مَاذَا يُنفِقُونَ قُلْ مَآ أَنفَقْتُم مِّنْ خَيْرٍ فَلِلْوَٰلِدَيْنِ وَٱلْأَقْرَبِينَ وَٱلْيَتَٰمَىٰ وَٱلْمَسَٰكِينِ وَٱبْنِ ٱلسَّبِيلِ وَمَا تَفْعَلُوا۟ مِنْ خَيْرٍ فَإِنَّ ٱللَّهَ بِهِۦ عَلِيمٌ ﴿٢١٥﴾

Acts of charity are like sweet nectar that benefits the giver and the needy. Furthermore the psychological health benefits that a person receives from helping others are indeed great. If you suffer from anxiety or depression, acts of charity have more potent effect on your health than the best medicines. Even if you smile when you meet someone, you are giving charity. Every time you smile, you not only make other people feel better about themselves, but you raise your self-esteem, increase your level of positive attitude and feel better about yourself as well. The Messenger of Allah (peace and blessings be upon him) said: "Never dismiss certain acts of kindness by deeming them to be insignificant, even if such an act is to meet your brother with a smiling face, for that is a deed which might weigh heavily in your scale of deeds."

Most people understand that they smile when they feel happy and frown when they feel sad. But few know that when the facial muscles that are used to create a smile are activated it can generate feelings of happiness. On the other hand, when you frown due to sadness or anger, you are displaying a sign of bitterness, an act that is very harmful to your health and to everyone, and only God knows the full extent of its evil effects.

All who obey Allah and the messenger are in the company of those on whom is the Grace of Allah, of the prophets (who teach), the sincere (lovers of Truth), the witnesses (who testify), and the Righteous (who do good): Ah! What a beautiful fellowship! (Quran 4:69)

وَمَن يُطِعِ ٱللَّهَ وَٱلرَّسُولَ فَأُوْلَٰٓئِكَ مَعَ ٱلَّذِينَ أَنْعَمَ ٱللَّهُ عَلَيْهِم مِّنَ ٱلنَّبِيِّـۧنَ وَٱلصِّدِّيقِينَ وَٱلشُّهَدَآءِ وَٱلصَّٰلِحِينَ وَحَسُنَ أُوْلَٰٓئِكَ رَفِيقًا ۝

And keep yourself patient [by being] with those who call upon their Lord in the morning and the evening, seeking His countenance. And let not your eyes pass beyond them, desiring adornments of the worldly life, and do not obey one whose heart We have made heedless of Our remembrance and who follows his desire and whose affair is ever [in] neglect. (Quran 18:28)

وَٱصْبِرْ نَفْسَكَ مَعَ ٱلَّذِينَ يَدْعُونَ رَبَّهُم بِٱلْغَدَوٰةِ وَٱلْعَشِيِّ يُرِيدُونَ وَجْهَهُۥ ۖ وَلَا تَعْدُ عَيْنَاكَ عَنْهُمْ تُرِيدُ زِينَةَ ٱلْحَيَوٰةِ ٱلدُّنْيَا ۖ وَلَا تُطِعْ مَنْ أَغْفَلْنَا قَلْبَهُۥ عَن ذِكْرِنَا وَٱتَّبَعَ هَوَىٰهُ وَكَانَ أَمْرُهُۥ فُرُطًا ۝

Hadith on Animals:

Allah forgave a prostitute for her kindness to thirsty dog

The Messenger of Allah (peace and blessings be upon him) said: "A Jewish prostitute had once been forgiven. She passed by a dog panting near a well. Thirst had nearly killed him, so she took off her sock, tied it to her veil, and drew up some water. Allah forgave her and He rewarded her for that deed with Paradise, which is as wide as the earth, the stars, and the heavens."

This is because Allah, the Giver of rewards, is the most Forgiving, Rich, and Worthy of Praise. O' you who are threatened by illness, fear and grief, occupy yourself in ways that are very useful to others. Help and support others through charity, sympathy, and hospitality.

And in doing so, you will find all of the richness and happiness that you desire. Those who criticize the contributors among the believers concerning [their] charities and [criticize] the ones who find nothing [to spend] except their effort, so they ridicule them - Allah will ridicule them, and they will have a painful punishment. (Quran 9:79)

ٱلَّذِينَ يَلْمِزُونَ ٱلْمُطَّوِّعِينَ مِنَ ٱلْمُؤْمِنِينَ فِي ٱلصَّدَقَٰتِ وَٱلَّذِينَ لَا يَجِدُونَ إِلَّا جُهْدَهُمْ فَيَسْخَرُونَ مِنْهُمْ سَخِرَ ٱللَّهُ مِنْهُمْ وَلَهُمْ عَذَابٌ أَلِيمٌ ﴿٧٩﴾

Repel depression, boredom through charity

Repel depression and boredom assisting people less fortunate than yourself. And in doing so, you will find all of the happiness that you seek. People spend their time gossiping and spreading rumors because their thoughts and minds are not at peace. Idleness allows your brain to drift into the pains of the past, the uncertainties of tomorrow and the future, and the difficulties of the present. So do rewarding work instead of feeling useless and helpless. Idleness is a veiled form of suicide, so save yourself. Our Lord, do not impose blame upon us if we have forgotten or erred. Our Lord, and lay not upon us a burden like that which You laid upon those before us. Our Lord, and burden us not with that which we have no ability to bear. And pardon us; and forgive us; and have mercy upon us. (Quran 2:286)

Idleness is a form of theft. One should always try to find something to do to provide for one's own and to share with those in need. Idleness is like torture.

It is slow and very painful. The Communist Chinese utilizes such torture to steal the souls of the people. Prisoners are placed under a bamboo tube from which a droplet of water falls only after every hour. During that period of waiting between drops of water, the broken prisoners lose their minds and are driven to insanity. May Allah rescue everyone from their evil. This world's life is naught but play and idleness and certainly the abode of the here-after is better for those who guard (against evil); do you not then understand? (Quran 6:32)

وَمَا ٱلْحَيَوٰةُ ٱلدُّنْيَآ إِلَّا لَعِبٌ وَلَهْوٌ وَلَلدَّارُ ٱلْأَخِرَةُ خَيْرٌ لِّلَّذِينَ يَتَّقُونَ أَفَلَا تَعْقِلُونَ ﴿٣٢﴾

Being inactive and lazy means being neglectful of one's responsibilities and duties. Idleness is an expert burglar and your brain and family are its victim. Stand up and say a prayer, read God's book, study, write a letter to a friend that you have seen in a long time, fix what is broken, or help others. Kill the boredom by doing something good. When you apply this simple advice, you will have traveled at least 65% of the way towards contentment. Look at farmers, bakers, carpenters, factory workers, and observe and witness how, when they are working, they remember Allah and they recite his phrases as melodious as the song of a nightingale, because they are very content and happy.

Do not be a imitate others

The Jewish people said: "Ezra is the son of Allah," and the Christians said: "The Messiah is the son of Allah." That is their statement from their mouths;

they imitate the saying of those who disbelieved [before them]. Exalted is He above having a son. To Him belongs whatever is in the heavens and whatever is on the earth. (Quran 9:30)

وَقَالَتِ ٱلۡيَهُودُ عُزَيۡرٌ ٱبۡنُ ٱللَّهِ وَقَالَتِ ٱلنَّصَٰرَى ٱلۡمَسِيحُ ٱبۡنُ ٱللَّهِۖ ذَٰلِكَ قَوۡلُهُم بِأَفۡوَٰهِهِمۡۖ يُضَٰهِـُٔونَ قَوۡلَ ٱلَّذِينَ كَفَرُواْ مِن قَبۡلُۚ قَٰتَلَهُمُ ٱللَّهُۚ أَنَّىٰ يُؤۡفَكُونَ ۝

Do not transform yourself into a disbeliever. Do not mimic others. From Prophet Adam (peace be upon him) to the last born person, no two humans are exactly the same. You are unique. None was like you in the past, and none will be exactly like you ever. Go forward according to your own nature. Always go onward according to your own nature and self. And [recall] when Moses prayed for water for his people, We said: "Strike with your staff the stone."

And there gushed forth from it twelve springs, and every people knew its watering place. (Quran 2:60) Twelve springs burst out of that stone, a designated spring for each tribe. Each tribe knew its place.

﴿ وَإِذِ ٱسْتَسْقَىٰ مُوسَىٰ لِقَوْمِهِۦ فَقُلْنَا ٱضْرِب بِّعَصَاكَ ٱلْحَجَرَ ۖ فَٱنفَجَرَتْ مِنْهُ ٱثْنَتَا عَشْرَةَ عَيْنًا ۖ قَدْ عَلِمَ كُلُّ أُنَاسٍ مَّشْرَبَهُمْ ۖ كُلُواْ وَٱشْرَبُواْ مِن رِّزْقِ ٱللَّهِ وَلَا تَعْثَوْاْ فِى ٱلْأَرْضِ مُفْسِدِينَ ﴾ ﴿٦٠﴾

And for every nation there is a direction to which they face (in their prayers). So hasten towards all that is good. Whosesoever you may be, Allah will bring you together (on the Day of Resurrection). Truly, Allah is Able to do all things. (Quran 2:148)

وَلِكُلٍّ وِجْهَةٌ هُوَ مُوَلِّيهَا ۖ فَٱسْتَبِقُواْ ٱلْخَيْرَٰتِ ۚ أَيْنَ مَا تَكُونُواْ يَأْتِ بِكُمُ ٱللَّهُ جَمِيعًا ۚ إِنَّ ٱللَّهَ عَلَىٰ كُلِّ شَىْءٍ قَدِيرٌ ﴿١٤٨﴾

Be as Allah had created you, and do not change your appearance, your voice, or modify your walk. The Messenger of Allah (peace and blessings be upon him) said: "Verily, Allah does not look at your appearance or wealth, but rather he looks at your hearts and actions." Enrich your heart and soul by following what is found in God's Book. Never try reduce yourself by imitating others and depriving yourself of your own uniqueness. The Messenger of Allah (peace and blessings be upon him) said: "And let no one amongst you be an imitator of others."

In terms of characteristics, we are like nature, with all its splendor and diversity of trees and plants: short and tall, bitter and sweet, colorful, and so on. Your value and worth is in being you, your natural self. People's different personalities, physical traits, languages, talents and abilities are signs from our Creator.

O mankind, indeed We have created you from male and female and made you from different tribes so that you may know one another. Indeed, the most noble of you in the sight of Allah is the most righteous of you. Indeed, Allah is Knowing and Acquainted. (Quran 49:13)

يَٰٓأَيُّهَا ٱلنَّاسُ إِنَّا خَلَقْنَٰكُم مِّن ذَكَرٍ وَأُنثَىٰ وَجَعَلْنَٰكُمْ شُعُوبًا وَقَبَآئِلَ لِتَعَارَفُوٓا۟ۚ إِنَّ أَكْرَمَكُمْ عِندَ ٱللَّهِ أَتْقَىٰكُمْۚ إِنَّ ٱللَّهَ عَلِيمٌ خَبِيرٌ ۝

Destiny preordained by Allah

No calamity befalls on the earth or in yourselves but is inscribed in the Book of Decrees (Al-Lauh Al-Mahfuz), before We bring it into existence. Verily, that is easy for Allah. . (Quran 57:22) This is a very important secret that underlies the testing by Allah that takes place in this world. Strong believers who possess this secret confront everything that befalls them with great patience and faith.

Muslims understand that the Creator has created all things within destiny and that what befalls a person does so solely because Allah so wishes. It is Allah Who creates all life, right down to the finest detail. Surat al-An'am tells us how everything, big or small, that happens occur only because Allah wishes it to happen: "The keys of the Unseen are in His possession. None knows them except Him. And He knows what is on the land and in the sea. Not a leaf falls but that He knows about it. And no grain is there within the darkness of the earth and no moist or dry [thing] but that it is [written] in a clear record." (Quran 6:59)

۞ وَعِندَهُۥ مَفَاتِحُ ٱلۡغَيۡبِ لَا يَعۡلَمُهَآ إِلَّا هُوَۚ وَيَعۡلَمُ مَا فِى ٱلۡبَرِّ وَٱلۡبَحۡرِۚ وَمَا تَسۡقُطُ مِن وَرَقَةٍ إِلَّا يَعۡلَمُهَا وَلَا حَبَّةٖ فِى ظُلُمَٰتِ ٱلۡأَرۡضِ وَلَا رَطۡبٖ وَلَا يَابِسٍ إِلَّا فِى كِتَٰبٖ مُّبِينٖ ۝

All human beings are constrained by time and by seeing events solely from the current instant. So since we do not know the future, we may not always be able to appreciate the long-term wisdom, beauty and goodness in events.

It is Allah who takes your souls by night and knows what you have committed by day. Then He revives, and to Him will be your return; then He will inform you about what you used to do. (Quran 6:60)

$$\text{وَهُوَ ٱلَّذِى يَتَوَفَّىٰكُم بِٱلَّيْلِ وَيَعْلَمُ مَا جَرَحْتُم بِٱلنَّهَارِ ثُمَّ يَبْعَثُكُمْ فِيهِ لِيُقْضَىٰٓ أَجَلٌ مُّسَمًّى ۖ ثُمَّ إِلَيْهِ مَرْجِعُكُمْ ثُمَّ يُنَبِّئُكُم بِمَا كُنتُمْ تَعْمَلُونَ ﴿٦٠﴾}$$

And He is the subjugator over His servants, and He sends over you guardian-angels until when death comes, then Our messengers take him, and they do not fail [in their duties]. (Quran 6:61)

$$\text{وَهُوَ ٱلْقَاهِرُ فَوْقَ عِبَادِهِۦ ۖ وَيُرْسِلُ عَلَيْكُمْ حَفَظَةً حَتَّىٰٓ إِذَا جَآءَ أَحَدَكُمُ ٱلْمَوْتُ تَوَفَّتْهُ رُسُلُنَا وَهُمْ لَا يُفَرِّطُونَ ۝}$$

Then they His servants are returned to Allah, their true Lord. Unquestionably, He is the destiny and judge, and He is the swiftest of accountants. (Quran 6:62)

$$\text{ثُمَّ رُدُّوٓا۟ إِلَى ٱللَّهِ مَوْلَىٰهُمُ ٱلْحَقِّ ۚ أَلَا لَهُ ٱلْحُكْمُ وَهُوَ أَسْرَعُ ٱلْحَاسِبِينَ ۝}$$

Allah is unfettered by time, so He sees and knows everything. Allah knows all these things that we cannot. The past, the future, and present are all one in the sight of Allah. All events are all already over and done with. However, we can only learn about them by going through them when the time comes. As revealed in the verse: No kind of calamity can occur, except by the leave of Allah: and if any one believes in Allah, (Allah) guides his heart (aright): for Allah knows all things. (Quran 64:11)

مَا أَصَابَ مِن مُّصِيبَةٍ إِلَّا بِإِذْنِ ٱللَّهِ وَمَن يُؤْمِنۢ بِٱللَّهِ يَهْدِ قَلْبَهُۥ وَٱللَّهُ بِكُلِّ شَىْءٍ عَلِيمٌ ﴿١١﴾

And obey Allah and obey the Messenger; but if you turn away - then upon Our Messenger is only [the duty of] clear notification. (Quran 64:12) Believers enjoy the fact of knowing that everything befalling them is destined to do so.

وَأَطِيعُوا۟ ٱللَّهَ وَأَطِيعُوا۟ ٱلرَّسُولَ فَإِن تَوَلَّيْتُمْ فَإِنَّمَا عَلَىٰ رَسُولِنَا ٱلْبَلَٰغُ ٱلْمُبِينُ ﴿١٢﴾

As a great blessing, Allah has created the testing of His slaves to be very easy. But this ease only applies to true believers who resign themselves to destiny. A person who truly believes and sincerely submits themselves to Allah watches the constant change of images before them with joy, thanks, and gratitude. Someone sitting watches the destiny appointed for him with trust and pleasure.

The images of that fate, sometimes scary, but have been specially prepared for them. Allah plans everything right down to the finest detail. But at the end of each day, they are all under the control of the Master Creator, Allah.

A good believer knows that the moral values he/she displays in the face of such test are very appreciated in the sight of Allah. This is a pleasure unique only to true believers. You must never suffer feelings of worry, stress, or fear in the face of such difficulties. Because a good believer knows that Allah will make everything turn out well in the end. In one verse, Allah tells believers that He will never will give the disbelievers over the believers a way [to overcome them]. (Quran 4:141)

ٱلَّذِينَ يَتَرَبَّصُونَ بِكُمْ فَإِن كَانَ لَكُمْ فَتْحٌ مِّنَ ٱللَّهِ قَالُوٓا۟ أَلَمْ نَكُن مَّعَكُمْ وَإِن كَانَ لِلْكَافِرِينَ نَصِيبٌ قَالُوٓا۟ أَلَمْ نَسْتَحْوِذْ عَلَيْكُمْ وَنَمْنَعْكُم مِّنَ ٱلْمُؤْمِنِينَ ۚ فَٱللَّهُ يَحْكُمُ بَيْنَكُمْ يَوْمَ ٱلْقِيَامَةِ ۗ وَلَن يَجْعَلَ ٱللَّهُ لِلْكَافِرِينَ عَلَى ٱلْمُؤْمِنِينَ سَبِيلًا ۝١٤١

People may encounter all kinds of difficulties in this life. For example, they may lose the ability to walk, hear, or see. They may fall ill, die or be killed. Allah tests His servants and rewards them for the courage they display many times over in this world and the next. Then they are given the eternal life of the Hereafter. The words of the people that were tested before us are reported in the following verse: And why should we not rely upon Allah while He has guided us to our [good] ways. And we will surely be patient against whatever harm you should cause us. And upon Allah let those who would rely [indeed] rely. (Quran 14:12)

وَمَا لَنَآ أَلَّا نَتَوَكَّلَ عَلَى ٱللَّهِ وَقَدْ هَدَىٰنَا سُبُلَنَا ۚ وَلَنَصْبِرَنَّ عَلَىٰ مَآ ءَاذَيْتُمُونَا ۚ وَعَلَى ٱللَّهِ فَلْيَتَوَكَّلِ ٱلْمُتَوَكِّلُونَ ﴿١٢﴾

And those who disbelieved said to the messengers, "We will surely drive you out of our land, or you must return to our religion." So their Lord inspired to them, "We will surely destroy the wrongdoers. (Quran 14:13)

وَقَالَ ٱلَّذِينَ كَفَرُوا۟ لِرُسُلِهِمْ لَنُخْرِجَنَّكُم مِّنْ أَرْضِنَآ أَوْ لَتَعُودُنَّ فِى مِلَّتِنَا ۖ فَأَوْحَىٰٓ إِلَيْهِمْ رَبُّهُمْ لَنُهْلِكَنَّ ٱلظَّٰلِمِينَ ﴿١٣﴾

And We will surely cause you to dwell in the land after them. That is for he who fears My position and fears My threat. (Quran 14:14)

وَلَنُسْكِنَنَّكُمُ ٱلْأَرْضَ مِنۢ بَعْدِهِمْ ۚ ذَٰلِكَ لِمَنْ خَافَ مَقَامِى وَخَافَ وَعِيدِ ﴿١٤﴾

Say: "Never will we be struck except by what Allah has decreed for us; He is our protector." (Quran 9:51)

قُل لَّن يُصِيبَنَا إِلَّا مَا كَتَبَ ٱللَّهُ لَنَا هُوَ مَوْلَىٰنَا ۚ وَعَلَى ٱللَّهِ فَلْيَتَوَكَّلِ ٱلْمُؤْمِنُونَ ﴿٥١﴾

And upon Allah let the believers rely. So there is no doubt that all these things are the results of their trust and faith in Allah and their submission to the destiny created by Him. Everyone that places their trust in Allah should never feel fear or distress.

Indeed, those who have said: "Our Lord is Allah," and then remained on a right course - there will be no fear concerning them, nor will they grieve. (Quran 46:13)

إِنَّ ٱلَّذِينَ قَالُوا۟ رَبُّنَا ٱللَّهُ ثُمَّ ٱسْتَقَـٰمُوا۟ فَلَا خَوْفٌ عَلَيْهِمْ وَلَا هُمْ يَحْزَنُونَ ﴿١٣﴾

Whoever submits themselves completely to Allah while being a doer of good will have his reward with his Lord. And no fear will there be concerning them, nor will they grieve. (Quran 2:112)

بَلَىٰ مَنْ أَسْلَمَ وَجْهَهُ لِلَّهِ وَهُوَ مُحْسِنٌ فَلَهُ أَجْرُهُ عِندَ رَبِّهِ وَلَا خَوْفٌ عَلَيْهِمْ وَلَا هُمْ يَحْزَنُونَ ﴿١١٢﴾

Just know that the friends of Allah will feel no fear and will know no sorrow. Those who have iman (faith), there will be no fear concerning them, nor will they grieve. (Quran 10: 62-63).

أَلَا إِنَّ أَوْلِيَاءَ اللَّهِ لَا خَوْفٌ عَلَيْهِمْ وَلَا هُمْ يَحْزَنُونَ ﴿٦٢﴾ الَّذِينَ ءَامَنُوا وَكَانُوا يَتَّقُونَ ﴿٦٣﴾

For them are good tidings in the worldly life and in the Hereafter. No change is there in the words of Allah. That is what the great attainment is. (Quran 10:64)

$$\text{لَهُمُ ٱلْبُشْرَىٰ فِى ٱلْحَيَوٰةِ ٱلدُّنْيَا وَفِى ٱلْءَاخِرَةِ لَا تَبْدِيلَ لِكَلِمَٰتِ ٱللَّهِ ذَٰلِكَ هُوَ ٱلْفَوْزُ ٱلْعَظِيمُ ﴿٦٤﴾}$$

In next verse, Allah says that the servants who believe in and surrender themselves to Him are bound to a strong branch that will never break. And whoever submits his face to Allah while he is a doer of good - then he has grasped the most trustworthy handhold. And to Allah will be the outcome of [all] matters. (Quran 31:22)

$$\text{۞ وَمَن يُسْلِمْ وَجْهَهُۥٓ إِلَى ٱللَّهِ وَهُوَ مُحْسِنٌ فَقَدِ ٱسْتَمْسَكَ بِٱلْعُرْوَةِ ٱلْوُثْقَىٰ وَإِلَى ٱللَّهِ عَٰقِبَةُ ٱلْأُمُورِ ﴿٢٢﴾}$$

And whoever has disbelieved - let not his disbelief grieve you. To Us is their return, and We will inform them of what they did. Indeed, Allah is Knowing of that within the breasts. (Quran 31:23)

$$\text{وَمَن كَفَرَ فَلَا يَحْزُنكَ كُفْرُهُۥٓ ۚ إِلَيْنَا مَرْجِعُهُمْ فَنُنَبِّئُهُم بِمَا عَمِلُوٓا۟ ۚ إِنَّ ٱللَّهَ عَلِيمٌۢ بِذَاتِ ٱلصُّدُورِ ﴿٢٣﴾}$$

Those who push others to religion is wrong. There is no compulsion (force) where the deen (religion) is concerned. Say: "To Allah belongs the east and the west. He guides whom He wills to the straight path." (Quran 2:142)

$$\text{۞ سَيَقُولُ ٱلسُّفَهَآءُ مِنَ ٱلنَّاسِ مَا وَلَّىٰهُمْ عَن قِبْلَتِهِمُ ٱلَّتِى كَانُوا۟ عَلَيْهَا ۚ قُل لِّلَّهِ ٱلْمَشْرِقُ وَٱلْمَغْرِبُ ۚ يَهْدِى مَن يَشَآءُ إِلَىٰ صِرَٰطٍ مُّسْتَقِيمٍ ﴿١٤٢﴾}$$

So there shall be no compulsion in [acceptance of] the religion. The right course has become clear from the wrong. So whoever disbelieves in Satan and believes in Allah has grasped the most trustworthy handhold with no break in it. And Allah is Hearing and Knowing. (Quran 2:256)

لَآ إِكْرَاهَ فِى ٱلدِّينِ قَد تَّبَيَّنَ ٱلرُّشْدُ مِنَ ٱلْغَيِّ فَمَن يَكْفُرْ بِٱلطَّٰغُوتِ وَيُؤْمِنۢ بِٱللَّهِ فَقَدِ ٱسْتَمْسَكَ بِٱلْعُرْوَةِ ٱلْوُثْقَىٰ لَا ٱنفِصَامَ لَهَا ۗ وَٱللَّهُ سَمِيعٌ عَلِيمٌ ﴿٢٥٦﴾

Whomever seeks Allah on their own, Allah will love them and guide. And seek help through patience and prayer, and indeed, it is difficult except for the humbly submissive [to Allah] (Quran 2:45)

وَٱسْتَعِينُوا۟ بِٱلصَّبْرِ وَٱلصَّلَوٰةِ ۚ وَإِنَّهَا لَكَبِيرَةٌ إِلَّا عَلَى ٱلْخَٰشِعِينَ ﴿٤٥﴾

Allah's pen already wrote everything. All events that shall come have already been written. Say; "Never will we be struck except by what Allah has decreed for us; He is our protector." And upon Allah let the believers rely. (Quran 9:51)

$$\text{قُل لَّن يُصِيبَنَآ إِلَّا مَا كَتَبَ ٱللَّهُ لَنَا هُوَ مَوْلَىٰنَا ۚ وَعَلَى ٱللَّهِ فَلْيَتَوَكَّلِ ٱلْمُؤْمِنُونَ ۝}$$

So whatever has befallen you was never destined to escape you, and whatever escaped you was never destined to befall you. If you believe in this firmly, then all suffering and hardship would become ease and comfort. The Messenger of Allah (peace be upon him) said: "Whomever Allah wishes good for, He will test them (with hardship)." For this reason, never feel sad if you are afflicted with illness, the death of a daughter or son, or the loss of wealth.

Allah, the Wise, had already decreed such matters to occur and the decision is His, and His alone. Be patient and have faith and you shall be rewarded, and your sins shall be atoned for. For those that are afflicted with tragedies, glad tidings await them and a beautiful garden. He is not questioned about what He does, but they will be questioned. (Quran 21:23)

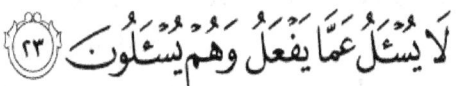

You will never feel comfort until you firmly trust that Allah has preordained all matters. His pen has already written everything that will happen to you. Allah has given everyone the free will and choice to do things and to refrain from others; to believe or disbelieve, and to obey or disobey. So Allah knows what you will do and what your ultimate destiny will be.

However, Allah never compels anyone to do evil, rather He clearly have shown everyone the path to take. He has sent Messengers and revealed Books to learn from. Whoever goes astray does so to his own loss. And say: "The truth is from your Lord, so whoever wills - let him believe; and whoever wills - let him disbelieve." Indeed, We have prepared for the wrongdoers a fire whose walls will surround them. And if they call for relief, they will be relieved with water like murky oil, which scalds [their] faces. Wretched is the drink, and evil is the resting place. (Quran 18:29)

وَقُلِ ٱلْحَقُّ مِن رَّبِّكُمْ فَمَن شَاءَ فَلْيُؤْمِن وَمَن شَاءَ فَلْيَكْفُرْ إِنَّا أَعْتَدْنَا لِلظَّٰلِمِينَ نَارًا أَحَاطَ بِهِمْ سُرَادِقُهَا وَإِن يَسْتَغِيثُوا يُغَاثُوا بِمَاءٍ كَٱلْمُهْلِ يَشْوِى ٱلْوُجُوهَ بِئْسَ ٱلشَّرَابُ وَسَاءَتْ مُرْتَفَقًا ﴿٢٩﴾

Some things are truly beyond our control. So never feel sorrow over that which is not in your hands.

For example, you could not have prevented the horse from falling, the wind from blowing, the flood from happening, or the dam from failing. You could not have prevented any of these things even if you tried. Surrender yourself to fate before anger and regret overwhelm you. All that has been preordained shall come to pass.

If you have tried your utmost, but still what you had been trying to prevent still occurred, then have faith that it was meant to happen. Never say: "If I had only done this it would have never happened." This is the decree of Allah. He cannot be questioned about what He does, but we will be questioned. So you see those in whose hearts is disease hastening into [association with] them, saying, "We are afraid a misfortune may strike us." But perhaps Allah will bring conquest or a decision from Him, and they will become, over what they have been concealing within themselves, regretful. (Quran 5:52)

فَتَرَى ٱلَّذِينَ فِى قُلُوبِهِم مَّرَضٌ يُسَٰرِعُونَ فِيهِمْ يَقُولُونَ نَخْشَىٰٓ أَن تُصِيبَنَا دَآئِرَةٌ فَعَسَى ٱللَّهُ أَن يَأْتِىَ بِٱلْفَتْحِ أَوْ أَمْرٍ مِّنْ عِندِهِۦ فَيُصْبِحُوا۟ عَلَىٰ مَآ أَسَرُّوا۟ فِىٓ أَنفُسِهِمْ نَٰدِمِينَ ﴿٥٢﴾

Allah brings victory or action according to His Will. The lost may find their way, the afflicted may find relief, and the fearful may find peace. Who, when afflicted with calamity, says: "Truly! To Allah we belong and truly, to Him we shall return," (Quran 2:156) Allah will say: "Build for My slave a house in Paradise and call it the house of praise."

ٱلَّذِينَ إِذَآ أَصَٰبَتْهُم مُّصِيبَةٌ قَالُوٓا۟ إِنَّا لِلَّهِ وَإِنَّآ إِلَيْهِ رَٰجِعُونَ ﴿١٥٦﴾

Those are the ones upon whom are blessings from their Lord and mercy. And it is those who are the [rightly] guided. (Quran 2:157)

$$\text{أُو۟لَـٰٓئِكَ عَلَيْهِمْ صَلَوَٰتٌ مِّن رَّبِّهِمْ وَرَحْمَةٌ ۖ وَأُو۟لَـٰٓئِكَ هُمُ ٱلْمُهْتَدُونَ ۝١٥٧}$$

If you are tired and lost, and you see that the hot desert extends for a thousand miles, just know that beyond that tiring distance is water and gardens with plentiful of shade. If you cannot breathe, and you feel a noose around your neck tightening and tightening, know that the rope will snap if you call out to him. He will respond.

And when My servants ask you, [O Muhammad], concerning Me - indeed I am near. I respond to the invocation of the supplicant when he calls upon Me. So let them respond to Me [by obedience] and believe in Me that they may be [rightly] guided. (Quran 2:186)

$$\text{وَإِذَا سَأَلَكَ عِبَادِى عَنِّى فَإِنِّى قَرِيبٌ ۖ أُجِيبُ دَعْوَةَ ٱلدَّاعِ إِذَا دَعَانِ ۖ فَلْيَسْتَجِيبُوا۟ لِى وَلْيُؤْمِنُوا۟ بِى لَعَلَّهُمْ يَرْشُدُونَ ۝١٨٦}$$

Do not lose hope in the mercy of Allah. Truly no one should despair of Allah's Mercy, except those who have no faith. If Allah should aid you, no one can overcome you. If you put your whole trust in Him, as you must, He will guide and satisfy your needs. Your tears will be followed by smiles, and your fear will be replaced by comfort and happiness. When Prophet Ibrahim (Abraham) (peace be and blessing be upon him) was thrown into the fire, he did not feel its heat, because if you believe that Allah stands with you, then it does not matter who stands against you. Allah said: "O fire, be coolness and safety upon Abraham." (Quran 21:69)

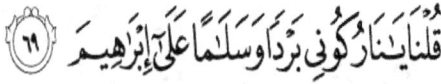

The Red Sea could not drown and swallow Prophet Moses (peace and blessings be upon him). He said: "No! Indeed, with me is my Lord. He will guide and protect me." (Quran 26:62)

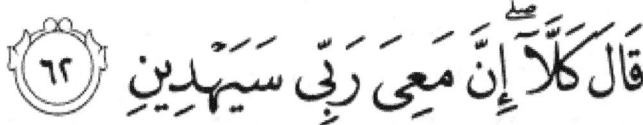

Then We inspired to Moses, "Strike with your staff the sea, and it parted, and each portion was like a great towering mountain. (Quran 26:63)

فَأَوْحَيْنَآ إِلَىٰ مُوسَىٰٓ أَنِ ٱضْرِب بِّعَصَاكَ ٱلْبَحْرَ ۖ فَٱنفَلَقَ فَكَانَ كُلُّ فِرْقٍ كَٱلطَّوْدِ ٱلْعَظِيمِ ۝

And We saved Moses and those with him, all together. (Quran 26:65)

وَأَنجَيْنَا مُوسَىٰ وَمَن مَّعَهُۥٓ أَجْمَعِينَ ۝

The Prophet (peace and blessings be upon him) preached to the people to trust in Allah. In the loneliness of Makkah, in the midst of persecution and danger, in adversity and tribulations, and when all enemies were around him, complete faith and trust in Allah was the dominant feature in his life.

However great the danger that confronted him, he (peace and blessings be upon him) never lost hope and never allowed himself to be unduly agitated. For example, when the Messenger of Allah (peace be upon him) was in the cave with Abu Bakr. Abu Bakr heard voices outside of the cave. The Prophet said" "Be not afraid, certainly Allah is with us."

Allah aided them when those who disbelieved had driven them out [of Makkah] as one of two, when they were in the cave and he said to his companion, "Do not grieve; indeed Allah is with us." And Allah sent down his tranquility upon him and supported him with angels you did not see and made the word of those who disbelieved the lowest, while the word of Allah - that is the highest. And Allah is Exalted in Might and Wise. (Quran 9:40)

$$\text{إِلَّا تَنصُرُوهُ فَقَدْ نَصَرَهُ اللَّهُ إِذْ أَخْرَجَهُ الَّذِينَ كَفَرُوا ثَانِيَ اثْنَيْنِ إِذْ هُمَا فِي الْغَارِ إِذْ يَقُولُ لِصَاحِبِهِ لَا تَحْزَنْ إِنَّ اللَّهَ مَعَنَا ۖ فَأَنزَلَ اللَّهُ سَكِينَتَهُ عَلَيْهِ وَأَيَّدَهُ بِجُنُودٍ لَّمْ تَرَوْهَا وَجَعَلَ كَلِمَةَ الَّذِينَ كَفَرُوا السُّفْلَىٰ ۗ وَكَلِمَةُ اللَّهِ هِيَ الْعُلْيَا ۗ وَاللَّهُ عَزِيزٌ حَكِيمٌ ﴿٤٠﴾}$$

When fear overwhelms, those that are slaves of that moment see only grief and despair. Do not lose courage. Be patient. Truly, Allah is with the patient. Therefore do not be in despair. It is impossible for time to stand still, for things to remain the same. If Allah should aid you, no one can overcome you. (Quran 3:160)

$$\text{إِن يَنصُرْكُمُ اللَّهُ فَلَا غَالِبَ لَكُمْ ۖ وَإِن يَخْذُلْكُمْ فَمَن ذَا الَّذِي يَنصُرُكُم مِّن بَعْدِهِ ۗ وَعَلَى اللَّهِ فَلْيَتَوَكَّلِ الْمُؤْمِنُونَ ﴿١٦٠﴾}$$

The seconds, minutes, hours, days, weeks, months, and years move on differently. The future is unseen, and every day Allah has matters to bring forth. And verily, with hardship there is relief. (Quran 94:5)

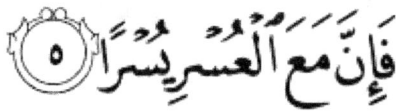

Verily, with the hardship, there is relief (i.e. there is one hardship with two reliefs, so one hardship cannot overcome two reliefs). (Quran 94:6)

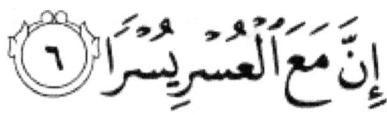

Turn lemons into sweet lemonade

The greater your storm, the brighter your rainbow. Trust in Allah! So transform losses into happiness. The Prophet (peace be upon him) was compelled to leave Makkah, however, he did not quit the Message of Allah. He continued it in Madinah. Allah closes doors, which no one can open and He opens doors, which no one can close. Imam Ahmad was severely tortured, and yet he did not give up. He became the Imam of the Sunnah. Imam Ibn Taymiyah was put into prison several times. He became a published scholar while behind bars. He wrote all his books during the seven years he spent in prison, except the book of Al-Eemaan, (The Faith) which he wrote in Egypt. Imam As-Sarakhsi was put in prison and kept at the bottom of a well. But he had strong faith. If Allah can turn night into day, then surely Allah can turn the darkness into happiness. So even at the bottom of the dark well, he wrote twenty volumes on Islamic jurisprudence.

Hafiz Ibn Kathir, became crippled and bind, but he still wrote many beautiful books. Imam Ibn al-Jawzi was thrown out his city and home, but through his travels, he became very proficient in the seven recitations of the Quran. Malik ibn ar-Rayb was on his deathbed when he wrote the most beautiful poem, which is loved till this day. So put your complete trust in Allah and believe there is nothing too hard for Him.

When you are tested with hardship and misfortune, be patient. If life handed you a glass full of squeezed sour lemons, be patient and add to it a handful of sugar. And if life gave you a snake as a gift, release it. Never give up hope in the mercy of Allah. Truly no one despairs of Allah's Mercy except those who have no faith. [Quran, 12:87]

يَـٰبَنِىَّ ٱذْهَبُوا۟ فَتَحَسَّسُوا۟ مِن يُوسُفَ وَأَخِيهِ وَلَا تَا۟يْـَٔسُوا۟ مِن رَّوْحِ ٱللَّهِ ۖ إِنَّهُۥ لَا يَا۟يْـَٔسُ مِن رَّوْحِ ٱللَّهِ إِلَّا ٱلْقَوْمُ ٱلْكَـٰفِرُونَ ﴿٨٧﴾

And it may be that you dislike a thing that is good for you. (Quran 2:216)

كُتِبَ عَلَيْكُمُ ٱلْقِتَالُ وَهُوَ كُرْهٌ لَّكُمْ ۖ وَعَسَىٰٓ أَن تَكْرَهُواْ شَيْـًٔا وَهُوَ خَيْرٌ لَّكُمْ ۖ وَعَسَىٰٓ أَن تُحِبُّواْ شَيْـًٔا وَهُوَ شَرٌّ لَّكُمْ ۗ وَٱللَّهُ يَعْلَمُ وَأَنتُمْ لَا تَعْلَمُونَ ۞

When the Romans destroyed Jerusalem, they jailed two great poets: one a pessimist and the other an optimist. In no time, both were able to squeeze their heads through the iron bars of the outside window. The optimist then looked at the stars and smiled, while the pessimist looked at the ground and dirt and wept.

Always take a look at the other side of any tragedy. A situation of truly pure evil never exists, and in all circumstances you can find some goodness and profit from a reward from the Creator.

Is He not best who responds to the desperate one when he calls upon Him and removes evil and makes you inheritors of the earth? Is there a deity with Allah? Little do you remember. (Quran 27:62)

أَمَّن يُجِيبُ ٱلْمُضْطَرَّ إِذَا دَعَاهُ وَيَكْشِفُ ٱلسُّوٓءَ وَيَجْعَلُكُمْ خُلَفَآءَ ٱلْأَرْضِ ۗ أَءِلَٰهٌ مَّعَ ٱللَّهِ ۚ قَلِيلًا مَّا تَذَكَّرُونَ ۝

From Whom do the hungry, the weak, and the oppressed seek victory? Who does everyone ask for help? He is Allah! Never give up hope in the mercy of Allah. Truly no one despairs of Allah's Mercy except those who have no faith. Therefore, it is important for you to ask for His help during times of both hardship and ease, to seek shelter with Him in most trying and difficult times, and to cry at His doorstep with tears of repentance and gratitude, then will His help and relief quickly arrive.

Rely upon Allah. Indeed, Allah loves those who rely [upon Him]. (Quran 3:159) If Allah should aid you, no one can overcome you; but if He should forsake you, who is there that can aid you after Him? And upon Allah let the believers rely. (Quran 3:160)

إِن يَنصُرْكُمُ ٱللَّهُ فَلَا غَالِبَ لَكُمْ ۖ وَإِن يَخْذُلْكُمْ فَمَن ذَا ٱلَّذِى يَنصُرُكُم مِّنۢ بَعْدِهِۦ ۗ وَعَلَى ٱللَّهِ فَلْيَتَوَكَّلِ ٱلْمُؤْمِنُونَ ﴿١٦٠﴾

He will save the one who is drowning. He will give victory to the oppressed and weak. He will guide the misguided and lost. He will cure the sick if they ask for His help, and He will provide relief to the afflicted and tired.

And when they board a ship, they supplicate Allah, sincere to Him in religion. But when He delivers them to the land, at once they associate others with Him. (Quran 29:65)

فَإِذَا رَكِبُوا۟ فِى ٱلْفُلْكِ دَعَوُا۟ ٱللَّهَ مُخْلِصِينَ لَهُ ٱلدِّينَ فَلَمَّا نَجَّىٰهُمْ إِلَى ٱلْبَرِّ إِذَا هُمْ يُشْرِكُونَ ﴿٦٥﴾

Say, "It is Allah who saves you from it and from every distress; then you [still] associate others with Him. (Quran 6:64)

قُلِ ٱللَّهُ يُنَجِّيكُم مِّنْهَا وَمِن كُلِّ كَرْبٍ ثُمَّ أَنتُمْ تُشْرِكُونَ ﴿٦٤﴾

As for the prayers one makes to remove hardship, recite the following prayer the Prophet (peace and blessing be upon him) made during a difficult time. When the persecution of Qurayish intensified following the death of his uncle and his wife, the Prophet (peace be upon him) went to the tribe of At-Taif, hoping that would listen to him and support him. But they rejected him and told their children to throw rocks at him until blood flowed to his body and feet.

The Prophet (peace be upon him) sought refuge in one of the gardens of At-Taif, and then he said the following beautiful and humble prayer to Allah:

اَللّٰهُمَّ اِلَيْكَ اَشْكُوْ ضَعْفَ قُوَّتِىْ وَقِلَّةَ حِيْلَتِىْ وَهَوَانِىْ عَلَى النَّاسِ يَاۤ اَرْحَمَ الرَّاحِمِيْنَ اَنْتَ رَبُّ الْمُسْتَضْعَفِيْنَ وَاَنْتَ رَبِّىْ اِلٰى مَنْ تَكِلُنِىْ اِلٰى بَعِيْدٍ يَتَجَهَّمُنِىْ اَمْ اِلٰى عَدُوٍّ مَلَّكْتَهُ اَمْرِىْ اِنْ لَمْ يَكُنْ بِكَ عَلَىَّ غَضَبٌ فَلَا اُبَالِىْ وَلٰكِنَّ عَافِيَتَكَ هِىَ اَوْسَعُ لِىْ اَعُوْذُ بِنُوْرِ وَجْهِكَ الَّذِىْ اَشْرَقَتْ لَهُ الظُّلُمَاتُ وَصَلُحَ عَلَيْهِ اَمْرُ الدُّنْيَا وَالْاٰخِرَةِ مِنْ اَنْ تُنْزِلَ بِىْ غَضَبَكَ اَوْ يَحِلَّ عَلَىَّ سَخَطُكَ لَكَ الْعُتْبٰى حَتّٰى تَرْضٰى وَلَا حَوْلَ وَلَا قُوَّةَ اِلَّا بِكَ

"O'Allah, to You do I complain of my weakness, little resource and lowliness before men. O'Most Merciful of those who show mercy, You are the Lord of the weak and You are my Lord. To whom will You leave me? To a far-off stranger who will mistreat me? Or to an enemy to whom You have granted power over me?

If You are not angry with me, then I care not, but Your favor is better for me. I seek refuge in the Light of Your Countenance by which the darkness is illumined and the things of this world and the next are set aright, lest Your anger descend upon me, or Your wrath light upon me. It is You Whom we beseech until You are well pleased. There is no power, and no strength except in You."

As for the various supplications one makes to remove hardship. I refer you to the books of the Sunnah. In them, you will learn prophetic supplications with which you can call to Allah supplicate to Him, and seek His aid. If you have found Him, then you have found everything. And if you lose your faith in Him, then you have lost everything. By supplicating to Him you are performing one of the highest forms of worship.

If you are persistent and sincere in your supplication, you will achieve freedom from worry and anxiety. All ropes are cut loose save His, and all doors are shut save His. He is near; He hears all and answers those who supplicate to Him. If you are living through affliction and pain, remember Allah, call out His name, and ask Him for help. Place your forehead on the ground and mention His praises, so that you can obtain true freedom. Raise your hands in supplication, and ask of Him constantly. Cling to His door, have good thoughts about Him, and wait for His help- you will then find true happiness and success.

Enough for you is your home

The words 'isolation' and 'seclusion' have a special meaning in our religion: to stay away from evil and its perpetrators, and to keep those who are foolish at a distance.

When you seclude yourself from evil in this manner, you will have an opportunity to reflect, to think, to graze in the meadows of enlightenment. When you isolate yourself from things that divert you from Allah's obedience, you are giving yourself a dose of medicine, one that doctors of the heart have found to be a most potent cure. When you seclude yourself from evil and idleness, your brain is stimulated into action. The results are increases in faith, repentance, and remembrance of Allah, the Most Merciful. However, some gatherings are not only recommended, but necessary, the congregational prayer, circles of learning, and all gatherings of righteousness. As for gatherings wherein frivolity and shallowness prevail, be wary of them. Take flight from such gatherings, weep over your wrongdoing, hold your tongue, and be content within the boundaries of your home.

By mixing with others based on foolish motives, you endanger the stability and soundness of your mind, for the people you indiscriminately mix with are likely to be experts at wasting time, masters at spreading lies, and skilled in spreading both trouble and mischief. Had they marched out with you, they would have added to you nothing except disorder, and they would have hurried about in your midst [spreading corruption] and sowing sedition among you... (Quran 9:47) I advise you to fortify yourself to your purpose and isolate yourself in your room, except when you leave it to speak well or to do well. When you apply this advice, you will find that your heart has returned to you. So use your time well and save your life from being wasted. Hold your tongue from backbiting free your heart from anxiety, and preserve your ears from profanity.

Your recompense is with Allah

When Allah takes something away from you. He compensates you with something better, but only if you are patient and seek your reward from Him. The Prophet (pbuh) said: "Whoever has his eyesight taken away from him and is (then) patient, he will be compensated for it with Paradise."

The Prophet (pbuh) said in another hadith: "Whoever loses a loved one from the people of this world and then seeks his recompense with his Lord, will be compensated with Paradise."

So do not feel excessive sorrow over some misfortune, because the One Who decreed it has with Him Paradise: recompense and a great reward. Those that are afflicted in this world and are close to Allah will be praised in the highest part of heaven. Peace be upon you, because you persevered in patience! Excellent indeed is the final home! (Quran 13:24)

Truly, the life of this world is short and its treasures are few. The Hereafter is better and everlasting, and whosoever is afflicted here shall find his reward there. And whosoever works hard here shall find ease there. As for those who cling to this world, who are attached to it, and who are in love with it, the hardest thing for them to bear would be to lose the world's comforts and riches: they desire to enjoy this life alone. Because of this desire, they don't react to misfortune as well as others do. What they perceive around them is this life alone: they are blind to its impermanence and insignificance. O' afflicted ones, if you are patient you lose nothing, and though you may not perceive it, you are profiting. The person who is afflicted with hardship should reflect upon the outcome in the Hereafter, the outcome for those who are patient.

Faith is life itself

Those that are wretched, in the full sense of the word, are those that are bereft of the treasures of faith. They are always in a state of misery and anger. The only means of purifying the heart and of removing anxieties and worries from it is to have complete faith in Allah, Lord of all that exists. In fact, there can be no true meaning to life when one has no faith. The best course of action that a confirmed atheist can take, if he will not believe is to take his own life. At least by doing so, he will free himself from the darkness and wretchedness in which he lives. How base and mean is a life without faith! How eternally accursed is the existence enveloping those who are outside of the boundaries set down by Allah! In proportion to the level of your faith -strong or weak, firm or wavering - will you be happy and at peace.

Whoever works righteousness, whether male or female, while he is a true believer, We shall pay them certainly a reward in proportion to the best of what they used to do [i.e. Paradise in the Hereafter]. (Quran 16:97)

People who lead this 'good life' will also have calm nerves when afflicted with hardship; they will be satisfied with everything that befalls them because it was written for them, and because they are pleased with Allah as their Lord, with Islam as their Religion, and with Muhammad as their Prophet and Messenger.

Extract the honey but do not break the hive

Everything that has gentleness in it is beautified, and whatever lacks it is spoiled. When you meet someone giving him a bright smile and a kind word, you are displaying a characteristic of the truly successful man a characteristic that even a bee exhibits. When a bee lands on a flower (doing so for a practical purpose) it does not destroy it, because Allah rewards gentleness with that which He does not give for harshness. There are certain people whose personalities are like magnets, attracting everyone who is nearby, simply because they are loved for their gentle talk their good manners, and their noble deeds. Winning the friendship of others is an art that is mastered by those that are noble and pious; a circle of people constantly surrounds them. Their mere presence in a gathering is a blessing, and when they are absent they are missed and asked about.

They suck out malice from others with their sincerity, forgiveness, and gentleness. They forget evil that was enacted upon them and preserve the memory of kindnesses received. Biting harsh words may be aimed at them but such words pass by their ears without entering and continue on their path without ever returning. They are in a state of calmness. People in general, and Muslims in particular, are safe from suffering any harm at their hands. The Prophet (Blessings and Peace be upon him) said: "The Muslim is the person whose tongue and hand do not harm other Muslims. And the Believer is he whom others trust with their blood and wealth."

Those who repress anger, and who pardon men; verily, Allah loves the gooddoers. (Quran 3:134)

Verily, in the remembrance of Allah do hearts find rest

Verily, in the remembrance of Allah do hearts find rest. (Quran 13:28) Truthfulness is beloved by Allah and is purifying g soap for the heart. And there is no deed that gives such pleasure to the heart, or has greater reward than the remembrance e of Allah. Therefore remember Me and I will remember you. (Quran 2:152)

Remembrance of Allah is His paradise on earth, and whoever does not enter it will not enter the Paradise of the Hereafter. Remembrance is not only a safe haven from the problems and worries of this world, but it is also the short and easy path to achieving ultimate success. Read the various revealed texts that refer to the remembrance of Allah, and you will appreciate its benefits.

When you remember Allah, clouds of worry and fear are driven away, and the mountains that make up your problems are blown away. We should not be surprised when we hear that people who remember Allah are at peace. What is truly surprising is how the negligent and unmindful survive without remembering Him.

To the degree that you remember Allah, your heart will be calm and cheerful. His remembrance carries with it the meaning of total dependence upon Him, of turning to Him for aid, of having good thoughts about Him, and of waiting for victory from Him. Truly, He is near when supplicated: He hears when He is called and He answers when He is invoked, so humble yourself before Him and ask of Him sincerely. Repeat His beautiful blessed name, and mention Him as being alone worthy of worship.

Mention His praises supplicate to Him, and ask forgiveness from Him: you will then find- by the will of Allah - happiness peace, and illumination. Jealousy is a disease that wreaks havoc not only on the mind, but also on the body. It is said that there is no repose for the jealous one and that he is an enemy wearing the garb of a friend. In doing justice to the disease of jealousy one can say that it is a fair one, for it begins with its bearer, killing him first. I forbid both you and myself from jealousy, because before we can show mercy to others we must first show it to ourselves. By being jealous of others, we are feeding misery with our flesh and blood and we are giving our sound sleep to others. The jealous person lights a fire and then jumps into it. Jealousy begets grief, pain, and suffering, thus destroying what was once a calm and virtuous life. The curse of the jealous one is that he contests fate and contends that his Creator is unjust.

How like a disease is jealousy, yet unlike other diseases -the one afflicted by it receives no reward in the Hereafter. The jealous person shall remain in fury until the day he dies, or until the good fortune of others departs from them. Everyone can be reconciled except the jealous one, because reconciliation with him requires that the blessings of Allah are removed from you or that you give up your talents and good qualities. If you were to do this, then perhaps he would become happy despite himself. We seek refuge in Allah from the evil of the jealous one, a person who becomes like a black poisonous snake, finding no repose until it releases its venom into an innocent body.

Accept life as it is

The pleasures of life are short-lived, and more often than not they are followed by sorrow. Life means responsibility, a journey wherein change is constant and difficulties are relentless in their onslaught. You will not find a father, a wife, or a friend who is free from problems. Allah has willed for this world to be filled with two opposites: good and evil, righteousness and corruption happiness and misery. Thus goodness, uprightness, and happiness are for Paradise; evil, corruption, and misery are for the Fire. So live according to your reality without always envisioning the ideal life, one that is free from worry and toil. Accept life as it is and adapt accordingly to all circumstances. You will not find in this world such things as the flawless companion or the perfect situation because flawlessness and perfection are qualities that are foreign to this life.

It is necessary for us to make amends: to take what is easy and leave what is difficult; and very frequently, to overlook the faults and mistakes of others.

Find consolation by remembering the afflicted

Look around you, to the right and to the left. Do you not see the afflicted and the unfortunate? In every house there is mourning and upon every cheek run tears. How many tribulations and how many people persevere with patience? You are not alone in your troubles, which are few compared to those of others. How many sick people remain bedridden for years while suffering from unspeakable pain? How many have not seen the light of the sun for years due to their imprisonment, having knowledge of nothing but the four corners of their cell? How many men and women have lost their dear children in the prime of youth?

How many people are troubled or tormented? Find consolation with those that are worse off than you, know that this life is like a prison for the believer, an abode of grief and sadness. In the morning castles are bustling with inhabitants; then in an instant, disaster occurs, and they are empty and desolate. Life can be peaceful, the body in good health, wealth abundant, and children healthy; and yet in only a matter of days, poverty, death, separation, and sickness can all take their place. And you dwelt in the dwellings of men who wronged themselves, and it was clear to you how We had dealt with them. And We put forth [many] parables for you. (Quran 14:45)

You must adapt like the experienced camel, which manages, when necessary, to kneel upon a rock.

You must also compare your difficulties with the difficulties of those around you, and with those that have come before you: you should realize that you are in good shape relative to them, and that you have merely been pricked by tiny difficulties. So praise Allah for His kindness be thankful for what He has left for you, seek recompense from Him for what He has taken and seek consolation with those that are afflicted. You have a perfect example in the Prophet (pbuh). The entrails of a camel were placed upon his head; his feet bled ; his face was fractured; he was besieged in a mountain pass until he was forced to eat tree leaves; he was driven out of Makkah; his front tooth was broken in battle ; his innocent wife was accused of wrongdoing; seventy of his Companions were killed; he was bereaved of his son and of most of his daughters; he would tie a stone around his stomach to lessen the pangs of hunger ; and he was accused of being a poet, a magician, a soothsayer, a madman, and a liar -all at the same time. Yet Allah protected him throughout these severe trials and tribulations. Prophet Zachariah was killed, Prophet Yahiya (John) was slaughtered. Prophet Moussa (Moses) was afflicted with great trials, Prophet Ibrahim (Abraham) was thrown in the fire, (may peace be upon them all), and the Imams of righteousness followed them upon this path. 'Umar was assassinated. Many scholars of the past have been flogged, imprisoned, or tortured. Or think you that you will enter Paradise without such [trials] as came to those who passed away before you? They were afflicted with severe poverty, ailments and were shaken. (Quran 2:214)

The prayer, the prayer

O' you who believe! Seek help in patience and the Prayer. (Quran 2:153) If you are beset with fear and anxieties stand up right now and pray: your soul will find comfort and solace.

The prayer- as long as you perform it sincerely with a wakeful heart -is guaranteed to have this effect for you. Whenever the Prophet (pbuh) was afflicted with hardship, he would say: "O' Bilal! Give us comfort and call for the prayer."

The prayer was his joy and pleasure; it was the delight of his eye. I have read biographies of many righteous people, who would always turn to prayer when they were surrounded by difficulties and hardship, people who would pray until their strength, will, and resolution returned to them. The Prayer of Fear (which is performed during battle) was prescribed in situations wherein limbs are severed, skulls fly, and souls depart from their bodies- a time when strength and resolution can only be derived from heartfelt prayer.

By earnestly performing the five daily prayers we achieve the greatest of blessings: atonement for our sins and an increase in rank with our Lord. Prayer is also a potent remedy for our sicknesses, for it instills faith in our souls. As for those that keep away from the Mosque and away from prayer, for them are unhappiness, wretchedness, and an embittered life. By leaving your affairs to Allah, by depending upon Him, by trusting in His promise by being pleased with His decree, by thinking favorably of Him, and by waiting patiently for His help, you reap some of ·the greater fruits of faith and display the more prominent characteristics of the believer. When you incorporate these qualities into your character, you will be at peace concerning the future, because you will depend on your Lord for everything. As a result, you will find care, help, protection, and victory.

When Prophet Ibrahim (Abraham) was placed in the fire, he said, "Allah (Alone) is Sufficient for us, and he is the Best Disposer of affairs (for us)." Thereupon. Allah made the fire to be cool, safe, and peaceful for Ibrahim. When the Prophet Muhammad (pbuh) and his Companions were threatened by the impending attack of the enemy, they said words that are related in the first part of this verse: "Allah [Alone] is Sufficient for us, and He is the Best Disposer of affairs [for us]. No harm touched them. If you face your enemy and are alarmed, or if you fear the misdeeds of the oppressor, say aloud: "Allah Alone is sufficient for us, and He is the Best Disposer of our affairs."

To isolate yourself to the confines of your own room while passing the hours away with lethal idleness, is a certain path to self-destruction. Your room is not the only place in the world, and you are not the sole inhabitant of it.

Then why do you surrender yourself to misery and solitude? Traveling to different lands is an activity which doctors recommend, especially for those who are feeling downcast, constricted by the narrowness of their own rooms. Therefore go forth and find delight in traveling.

Patience is most fitting

Those who meet hardship with a strong bearing and a patient countenance are in the minority. But we must consider this, though it may seem obvious: if you or I will not be patient then what else is there for us to do? Do you have an alternative solution? Do you know of any provision that is better than patience? Those that achieve greatness have to surmount an ocean of difficulties and hardships before finally achieving success. Know that each time you escape a difficulty you will have to face another.

Through this constant conflict, you must arm yourself with patience and a strong trust in Allah. This is the way of the noble-minded: they face difficulties with firm resolution, and they wrestle hardship to the ground. Therefore be patient and know that your patience is only through Allah. Have the patience of one who is confident of forthcoming ease, of one who knows that there will be a good ending, and of one who seeks reward from his Lord, hoping, that by facing difficulties, he will find expiation for his sins. Have patience, no matter what the difficulty and no matter how dark the road ahead seem. For truly, with patience comes victory, and with difficulty relief follows close behind. After having read biographies of some successful people from the past, I became amazed at the amount of patience they displayed, at their ability to bear heavy burdens only to emerge as stronger human beings.

Hardship fell upon their heads like the lashing of freezing rain and yet they were as firm as mountains. And then, after a short time had passed, they were rewarded for their patience with success.

Do not carry the weight of the globe ton your shoulders

In a certain class of people there rages an internal war, one that doesn't take place on the battlefield but in one's bedroom one's office, one's own home. It is a war that results in ulcers or an increase in blood pressure. Everything frustrates these people: they become angry at inflation, furious because the rains came late, and exasperated when the value of their currency falls. They are forever perturbed and vexed no matter what the reason.

They think that every cry is against them. (Quran 63:4)

My advice to you is this: do not carry the weight of the globe on your shoulders. Let the ground carry the burden of those things that happen. Some people have a heart that is like a sponge, absorbing all kinds of fallacies and misconceptions. It is troubled by the most insignificant of matters it is the kind of heart that is sure to destroy its possessor. Those who are principled and are upon the true path are not shaken by hardship; instead, hardship helps to strengthen their resolve and faith. But the reverse is true for the weak-hearted: when they face adversity or trouble it is only their level of fear that increases. At a time of calamity, there is nothing more beneficial to you than having a brave heart. On the other hand, during the course of any given day, the coward slaughters himself many times with apprehensions and presentiments of impending doom. Therefore, if you desire for yourself a stable life, face all situations with bravery and perseverance.

Be more resolute than your circumstances and more ferocious than the winds of calamity. May mercy descend upon the weak-hearted, for how often it is that they are shaken by the smallest of tremors? As for those who are resolute, they receive help from their Lord and are confident of His promise. He sent down calmness and tranquility upon them... (Quran 48:18)

Do not be crushed by what is insignificant

Many are those that are distressed not by pressing matters of great import, but by minor trifles. Observe the Hypocrites and how tweak they are in their resolution. A band of them ask for permission of the Prophet [Muhammad] saying: Truly, our homes lie open [to the enemy]'. And they lay not open. They but wished to flee) (Quran 33:13) ' We fear lest some misfortune of a disaster may befall us. (Quran 5:52)

How wretched are the souls of such people! Their principal concerns are for their stomachs, cars, houses, and castles. They never once raise their eyes to a life of ideals and virtues; the extent of their knowledge is their cars, clothes, shoes, and food. Some people are distressed day and night, because of a disagreement with their spouse, son, or relative or because they have had to forbear criticism or because of some other trivial event. Such are the calamities of these people. They have no aspiration to higher principles or goals to keep them busy, and they have no noble ambition in their lives to an end for which they can strive day and night. It has been said, 'When water leaves a container, it is then filled with air'. Therefore reflect on that which gives you cause for concern or anxiety, and ask yourself this: does it merit your energies and toils?

This is an indispensable question because whatever it is that causes your anxiety, you are, with mind, flesh, and blood giving it energy and time. And if it does not merit your energy and time, you will have squandered a great deal of your most precious resources. Psychologists say that you should judge everything in proportion to its true value and then put it in its proper place. More truthful than this is the saying of Allah:

Indeed Allah has set a measure for all things. (Quran 65:3)

So give to each situation according to its size, weight, measure, and importance. And stay away from immoderation or from exceeding the proper bounds. Take from the example of the Prophet's Companions, whose sole concern was to give their pledge of allegiance under the tree and thus obtain the pleasure of Allah.

With them was a man whose concern was focused on a missing camel, a preoccupation that caused him to miss the pledge of allegiance -and consequently, he was deprived of the rewards that were reaped by the others. Be content with that which Allah has given you and you will be the richest of people. So hold that which I have given you and be of the grateful. (Quran 7:144)

Most Islamic scholars and pious Muslims of the early generations of Islam were poor; needless it is to say, then, that they did not have beautiful houses or nice cars. Yet, despite these disadvantages, they led fruitful lives, and they benefited mankind not by some miracle, but because they used all that they were given, and spent their time in the correct way. Hence they were blessed in their lives, their time, and their talents.

On the contrary, there are many people who have been bestowed with wealth, children, and all forms of blessings yet these blessings have been the very reason for their misery and ruin. They deviated from what their inborn instincts were telling them, namely, that material things are not everything. If you are a seeker of happiness, be satisfied with the looks Allah has favored you with, with your family situation, with the sound of your voice, with the level of your understanding, and with the amount of your salary. Certain educators go further than this by saying that you should imagine being contented with even less than you actually have now. Remind yourself of Paradise, which is as wide as are the Heavens and the Earth. If you are hungry in this world, if you are sad, ill or oppressed, remember the eternal bliss of Paradise. If you do this, then your losses are really profits and the hardships you face are really gifts. The most wise of people are those that work for the

Hereafter, because it is better and everlasting. And the most foolish of mankind are those that see this world as their eternal abode- in it reside all of their hopes. You will find such people to be the most grief-stricken of all when faced with calamity. They will be the most affected by worldly loss simply because they see nothing beyond the insignificant lives that they lead. They see and think only of this impermanent life. They wish for nothing to spoil them in their state of felicity. Were they to remove the veil of ignorance from their eyes, they would commune with themselves about the etenıal abode- its bliss, pleasures, and castles. They would listen attentively when they are informed through the Quran and the Sunnah about its description. Indeed that is the abode that deserves our attention and merits our striving and our toiling, so that we may achieve the best of it. Have we reflected at length about the description of the inhabitants of Paradise?

Illness does not befall them grief does not come near them, they die not they remain young, and their attire remains both perfect and clean. They are in a beautiful home. In Paradise is found that which no eye has seen, no ear has heard, and no human mind has imagined. The rider travels under a tree in Paradise for one hundred years and yet he still does not reach its end. The length of a tent in Paradise is sixty miles. Its rivers are constant its castles are lofty, and its fruits are not only close-by, but are also easily picked.

Both your conscience and your Religion demand that you be just, which means that you should neither exaggerate nor understate neither go into excess nor do too little. Whoever seeks happiness should be just, regardless of whether he is in an angry, a sad, or a joyful mood. Exaggeration in our dealings with others is unacceptable. The best course is the middle course. Whoever follows his desires will likely magnify the importance of any given situation, always making a big deal out of nothing. He will feel jealous y and malice toward others. Since he lives in a world of exaggeration and imagination, he will envisage everyone else to be against him, even to the extent that he feels others to be always conspiring to destroy him. Because of this, he lives under a dark cloud, constantly overcome by fear and apprehension. Living according to hearsay and superstition is prohibited in our Religion. More often than not, what you fear will happen in the future does not end up taking place. Here is something you should try: when you fear something, imagine that the worst possible outcome takes place, and then train yourself to feel prepared and contented with that outcome. If you do this, you will find that you have saved yourself from apprehensions and superstitions that would otherwise have caused you much grief.

Lend your attention to each matter in proportion to its importance. In any given situation do not exaggerate mountains from mole hills; rather, keep in mind your objectivity and fairness. Do not follow false suspicion or the deceitful illusion of the mirage but be balanced. Listen to the balance of love and hate as explained by the Prophet (Blessings and Peace be upon him): "Love the one who is beloved to you in due moderation for perhaps the day will come when you will abhor him. And hate the one whom you detest in due moderation for perhaps the day will arrive when you will come to love him."

Perhaps Allah will make friendship between you and those whom you hold as enemies. And Allah has power [over all things], and Allah is Oft-Forgiving, Most Merciful.   (Quran 60: 7)

Being sad is not encouraged in our religion

So do not become weak [against your enemy], nor be sad. (Quran 3:139) (And grieve not over them, and be not distressed because of what they plot) (Quran 16:12 7)

[Be not sad, surely **Allah is with you**!] (Quran 9:40)

Sadness enervates the soul's will to act and paralyzes the body into inactivity. Sadness prevents one from action instead of compelling one towards it. The heart benefits nothing through grief. The most beloved thing to the Devil is to make the worshipper sad in order to prevent him from continuing on his path. Allah the Exalted, says: Secret counsels [conspiracies] are only from Shaytaan [Satan], in order that he may cause grief to the believers. (Quran 58:10)

In the following hadith the Prophet (pbuh) said: "In a company of three, it is forbidden for two to hold secret counsel to the exclusion of the third since doing so will be a cause of sadness for him."

Contrary to what some believe (those who have an extreme ascetic bent), the believer should not seek out sadness, because sadness is a harmful condition that afflicts the soul. The Muslim must repel sadness and fight it in any way that is permissible in our Religion. Grief is coupled with anxiety in this hadith. The difference between the two is that if a bad feeling is related to what is going to happen in the future then one is feeling anxiety. And if the cause of this feeling concerns the past, then one is feeling grief. Both of them weaken the heart causing inactivity and a decrease in will power. Despite what has been mentioned above, grief may sometimes be both inevitable 3nd necessary. When they enter Paradise, its dwellers will say:

All the praises and thanks be to Allah, Who has removed from us [all] grief. (Quran 35:34)

This verse implies that they were afflicted with grief in this life, just as they were afflicted with other forms of hardship, both of which were out of their control. So whenever one is overcome by grief and there is no way to avoid it, one is rewarded because grief is a form of hardship, and the believer is rewarded for going through hardship. Nonetheless the believer must ward off grief with supplication and other practical means. Therefore the good kind of grief is that which stems from missing out an opportunity to do a good deed or from performing a sin. When one feels sad because he was negligent in fulfilling the rights of Allah, he shows a characteristic of a person who is on the right path. As for the hadith, "Whatever befalls the believer in terms of anxiety, hardship or grief, Allah will make it an atonement for (some of) his sins."

This indicates that grief is a trial with which the believer is afflicted, and through which some of his sins are atoned for. However, it does not indicate that grief is something to be sought after the believer should not seek out means of finding grief, thinking that he is performing an act of worship. If this were the case, then the Prophet (pbuh) would have been the first to apply this principle. But he didn't search out for misery; rather, his face was always smiling, his heart was content, and he was continually joyful.

As for the hadith of Hind, "He was continually sorrowful," it is considered to be unsubstantiated by scholars of hadith, because among its narrators is someone who is unknown. Not only is the hadith weak because of its chain of narrators; it is also weak because it is contrary to how the Prophet (pbuh) really was.

How could he have been continually in grief when Allah had informed him that he was forgiven for everything (guaranteeing his entry into Paradise) and had protected him from feeling grief over matters pertaining to this life: for example, Allah forbade him from feeling grief over the actions of the disbelievers? How could he have felt grief when all the time his heart was filled with the remembrance of Allah, and when he was at peace with Allah's promise? In fact, he was always pleasant and his teeth were always visible due to his constant smiles. Whoever delves deeply into his life will know that he came to remove falsehood and to eradicate anxiety, confusion, and grief. He came to free our souls from the tyranny of doubt, disbelief, confusion, and disorder. He came to save our souls from destruction. So many indeed are the favors that were bestowed upon mankind through him (Blessings and Peace be upon him).

And as for the alleged hadith, "Verily, Allah loves all sad hearts," the chain of its narrators is unknown, so it is not an authentic hadith, especially in view of the fact that the basic principles of our religion are contrary to its import. Even if we were to suppose the hadith to be authentic then its meaning would be that sadness is one of the hardships of life imposed upon the worshipper as a form of trial. And if the worshipper is tested by this trial, and if he perseveres through patience, then Allah loves him. As for those who have praised melancholy and have lauded its many virtues (while claiming that our religion encourages it) then they are very mistaken. In fact, every text from revelation that touches upon sadness forbids it and orders its opposite: namely, that we should be content with the mercy and blessings of Allah, and happy with that which has been sent with the Messenger of Allah (Blessings and Peace be upon him).

Those who incline towards extremes in asceticism also relate the following narration:

"If Allah loves one of his slaves, He makes that slave's heart that of a weeper. And if he hates one of his slaves, then he places a flute in his heart (thus making him constantly light and happy)."

First, we must note that this is an Israelite tradition which is claimed to be found in the Torah. Nevertheless it does have a correct meaning since, truly, the believer feels grief due to his sins and the evildoer is ever playful and frivolous, light and joyful. So if the hearts of the faithful grieve, then it is only due to opportunities lost in terms of righteous deeds or because of sins committed. This is contrary to the sadness of the evildoers, whose grief is caused by losing out on physical pleasure or worldly benefit. Their yearnings anxieties, and sadness are always for these ends and for nothing else.

In this verse, Allah says of his Prophet Israaeel (Israel): And the lost this sight because of the sorrow that he was suppressing. (Quran 12:84)

Here we are informed of his grief over losing his beloved son. Simply informing us about something does not in itself signify either approval or disapproval of that thing. The fact is that we have been ordered to seek refuge from sadness, as it is a heavy cloud that hangs above its victim, and is a barrier that prevents one from advancing to higher aims. There is no doubt that sadness is a trial and a hardship, and is in some ways similar to sickness. However, it is not a stage, level, or condition that the pious should actively seek out. You are required to seek the means of happiness and peace, to ask Allah to grant you a good life, one that gives you a clear conscience and a mind at peace. The achievement of this is an early reward a point that is underscored by the saying of some, "In this world is a paradise, and whoever does not enter it shall not enter the Paradise of the Hereafter." And we ask Allah to open our hearts to the light of faith, to guide our hearts to His straight path, and to save us from a miserable and wretched life.

Take a moment to reflect

Let us make these supplications, their purpose being to eliminate hardship, anxiety and grief: There is none worthy of worship except Allah the Lord of the Tremendous Throne. There is none worthy of worship except Allah the Lord of the Heavens, the Lord of the earth, and the Lord of the Noble Throne. O' Ever-Living, and O' One Who sustains and protects all that exists, there is none worthy of worship except You, and by our mercy do we seek Your aid."

"O' Allah, verily I am Your slave, the son of Your slaves ; my forelock is in Your hand, Your order concerning me will be executed and just is Your judgment upon me. I ask You by all of Your names that you have named Yourself with, have revealed in Your book, have taught to one of Your creation, or is in Your knowledge only (from the matters of the unseen) - make the Quran the spring of my heart, the light of my chest, the remover of my sadness, and the purge of my anxiety."

"O' Allah, I seek refuge in you from anxiety and grief, from inability and laziness, from avarice and cowardice, from being engrossed by debt, and from being overpowered by men."

Smile

Laughing moderately can act as a cure or as therapy for depression and sadness. It has a strong influence on keeping the soul light and the heart clear. Abu Darda' (may Allah be pleased with him) said, "I make it a practice to laugh in order to give rest and comfort to my heart. And the noblest of people. Muhammad (pbuh), would laugh, sometimes until his molars became visible."

Laughing is an efficacious way to achieve comfort and light-heartedness but keep in mind that, as in other things, you should not be immoderate.

The Prophet (Blessings and Peace be upon him) said:

"Do not laugh excessively, for verily, excessive laughter kills the heart."

What is called for is moderation.

"And if you smile in the face of your brother, then that is a form of charity."

So he, Suleiman smiled, amused by her speech. (Quran 27:19)

Also, when you laugh, you should not do so in a mocking or jeering fashion. The Arabs would hold in high esteem a person who was known for his smile and laughter. They believed this to be a sign of a generous personality and of a person who has a noble disposition and a clear mind. The truth is that the principles of Islam are based on moderation and on good measure, whether it is in matters of belief, worship manners, or conduct. Islam does not condone a rigid frowning expression, nor does it condone a constant playful giddiness; rather what it does promote is seriousness when it is called for, and a reasonable level of light-heartedness when it is called for.

The Prophet (Blessings and Peace be upon him) said: "Do not disparage (underestimate) any good deed (no matter how small it is), even if that deed was to meet your brother with a friendly countenance."

"People who are always smiling not only make their own lives more joyful, but what is more, they are more productive people in their work and have a greater ability to live up to their responsibilities. They are more prepared to face difficulties and to find expedient solutions for them. They are prolific workers who benefit themselves and others."

If I were given a choice between having status in society and plentiful money, and between having a happy, radiant, smiling self, I would choose the latter. For what is great wea1th if it begets misery? And what is high position if what comes with it is constant gloominess? And what good is the most beautiful wife if she transforms her house into a living hell? Much better than her- a thousand times at least - is a wife who has not reached such a pinnacle of beauty, but nonetheless has made her house a kind of paradise.

Consider this imagery: In a sense, the rose is smiling and so is the forest. The oceans, rivers, the sky, the stars and birds are all smiling. Similarly, the human being by his very nature is a smiling entity, were it not for those things that counteract this natural disposition, such as greed and selfishness, evils that contribute to his frowning. As such he is an anomaly and at odds with the natural harmony of all that surrounds him. Therefore the person whose heart is sullied cannot see things as they truly are. Every person sees the world through himself -through his actions, thoughts, and motives. So if our actions are noble, if our thoughts are pure, and if our motives are honorable then the spectacles through which we see the world will be clean, and the world will be seen by us as it really is - a beautiful creation. If the spectacles become dirty, and their lenses stained, then everything will seem to be black and morbid.

There are those souls that are able to turn everything into misery, whilst there are those that are able to derive happiness from the most difficult of circumstances. There is the woman whose eyes fall upon nothing but mistakes. Today is black because a piece of fine china broke or because the cook put too much salt in the food. Then she flares up and curses, and no one in the house escapes from her execrations. Then there is the man who brings misery upon his own self and, through his disposition heaps the same upon others. Any word that he hears he interprets in the worst possible way. He is affected gravely by the most insignificant of things that occur to him, or that have occurred to him through his actions. He is drawn into misery by profits lost by profits expected that went unrealized, and so on. The whole world from his perspective is black, and so he blackens it for those around him. Such people have much ability to over-exaggerate the trifles that occur to them.

Thus they make mountains out of molehill s. Their ability to do well is negligent, and they are never happy or content with that which they have, even if what they have is plenty. No matter how great their possession s, they will never feel any blessings from what they have.

Life is like an art or a science: it needs to be learned and cultivated. It is much better for a person to plant love in his life than to glorify money, using all his might to help it ease its way into his pocket or into his account. What is life when all its energies are exploited and used for the sole purpose of accumulating wealth an existence where no energy is directed towards the cultivation of beauty, splendor, and love? Most people do not open their eyes to the beauty of life, but open them only to gold or silver. They pass by a lush and luxuriant garden, a beautiful bed of roses, a flowing river, or a group of singing birds, yet they are unmoved by such scenes. All that moves them is the coming and going of money into or out of their pockets. Money is but a means to a happy life. They have reversed this fact, have sold their happy existence, and have made money to be an end in itself. Our body has been equipped with eyes to see beauty with, yet we have trained them to look on nothing but money. Nothing causes the soul or the face to frown more often and with more intensity than despondency. If you want to be a smiling person wage war with despondency and hopelessness. The door to opportunity is always open to you and to others, and so is the door to success. So indoctrinate your mind with hopes of prosperity in the future.

Blessed is the one who has a teacher that helps him to develop his natural abilities and broaden his horizons. The best teacher is the one that instills kindness and generosity into his pupil, and teaches that the noblest of pursuits that one can strive for, is to be a source of goodness to others, in accordance with one's abilities.

The soul should be like the sun, radiating light and hope. The heart should be filled with tenderness, virtue, benevolence, and a genuine love for spreading goodness to all those that are connected to it. The smiling soul sees difficulties, and loves to surmount them. When it sees problems, it smiles, reveling in the opportunity to solve and overcome them. The frowning soul, when faced with a problem magnifies it and belittles its own determination, while spending all its time justifying. It loves success in life, but is not willing to pay its price. On every path it sees a grinning lion. It waits only for gold to shower down upon it, or to chance upon some treasure in the ground.

Difficult things in life are only relative, for everything is difficult for the ordinary person, while there is no great difficulty for the remarkable person. While the remarkable person increases in worthiness by overcoming obstacles, the weak person increases in meanness by running away from them. Problems are comparable to a vicious dog. When it sees you scared or running away, it barks and follows in pursuit. However, when it sees your scorn, your lack of concern, and when you shine your eyes in its direction, it gives way and draws back. Furthermore, there is nothing more deadly than a feeling of inferiority, a feeling that makes its holder lose all faith in his adequacy. So when he embarks upon a project he is immediately doubtful of its completion or success and he acts accordingly by gratifying these doubts. Thus he fails. Having self-confidence is a noble virtue, and is a pillar of success in life. It is important to note, though, that there is a vast difference between conceitedness and confidence. Conceitedness means to rely upon a deceitful imagination and false pride. Confidence means to rely upon true abilities it means fulfilling responsibilities developing talents and organizational skills.

How much in need we indeed are of a smile, a friendly face, easy-going manners, and a gentle, generous soul. The Prophet said: "Verily, Allah has revealed to me that you should be humble, so that none of you should transgress upon another, and so that none of you should be arrogant and proud to another."

Smile - Pause to reflect

When you experienced sadness yesterday, your situation didn't get any better by you being sad. Your son failed in school, and you became depressed, yet did your depression change the fact that he failed? Your father passed away, and you became downhearted, yet did that bring him back to life? You lost your business, and you became saddened. Did this change your situation by transforming losses into profits?

Do not be sad: You became despondent due to a calamity, and by doing so, created additional calamities. You became depressed because of poverty and this only increased the bitterness of your situation. You became gloomy because of what your enemies said to you by entering into that mental state, you unwittingly helped them in their attack against you. You became sullen because you expected a particular misfortune, and yet it never came to pass. Do not be sad: Truly a large mansion will not protect you from the effects of depression; and neither will a beautiful wife, abundant wealth a high position or brilliant children.

Do not be sad: Sadness causes you to imagine poison when you are really looking at pure water, to see a cactus when you are looking at a rose, to see a barren desert when you are looking at a lush garden, and to feel that you are in an unbearable prison when you are living on a vast and spacious earth.

Do not be sad: You have the true Religion to live by, a house to live in, bread to eat, water to drink, clothes to wear, a wife to find comfort with; why then the melancholy?

The blessing of pain

Pain is not always a negative force and it is not something that you should always hate. At times a person benefits when he feels pain. You might remember that at times when you felt a lot of pain you sincerely supplicated and remembered Allah. When he is studying, the student often feels the pangs of heavy burden sometimes perhaps the burden of monotony, yet he eventually leaves this stage of life a scholar. He felt burdened with pain at the beginning but he shined at the end. The aches and pangs of passion the poverty and the scorn of others, the frustration and anger at injustices -these all cause the poet to write flowing and captivating verses.

This is because he himself feels pain in his heart in his nerves, and in his blood, and as a result he is able to infuse the same emotions, via his work, into the hearts of others. How many painful experiences did the best writers have to undergo, experiences that inspired brilliant works, works that posterity continues to enjoy and benefit from today. The student who 1ives the life of comfort and repose and who is not stung by hardships or who has never been afflicted with calamity will be an unproductive, lazy, and lethargic person.

Indeed the poet who knows no pain and who has never tasted any bitter disappointments will invariably produce heaps upon heaps of cheap words. This is because his words pour forth from his tongue and not from his feelings or emotion, and though he may comprehend what he has written his heart and body have not lived the experience.

More worthy and relevant to the aforementioned examples are the lives of the early believers, who lived during the period of revelation and who took part in the most important religious revolution that mankind has ever seen. Indeed, they had greater faith, nobler hearts, truthful tongues, and deeper knowledge than those that came after them: they had all of these because they lived through pain and suffering, both of which are necessary concomitants to great revolutions.

They felt the pains of hunger, of poverty, of rejection, of abuse, of banishment from home and country, of abandonment of all pleasures of the pains of wounds, and of death and torture. They were in truth chosen ones, the elite of mankind. They were models of purity, nobleness, and sacrifice.

That is because they suffer neither thirst nor fatigue, nor hunger in the Cause of Allah nor they take any step to raise the anger of disbelievers nor inflict any injury upon an enemy, but is written to their credit as a deed of righteousness. Allah wastes not the reward of the doers of good. (Quran 9:120)

There are many examples of those that prospered and achieved as a result of the suffering they experienced. Therefore do not become excessively anxious when you think of pain, and do not fear suffering. It might well be that through pain and suffering you will become stronger. And furthermore, for you to live with a burning and passionate heart that has been stung is purer and nobler than to live the dispassionate existence of a person who has a cold heart and a shortsighted outlook. But Allah was averse to their being sent forth, so He made them lag behind, and it was said [to them], "Sit you among those who sit [at home]." (Quran 9:46)

The words of a passionate sermon can reach the innermost depths of the heart and penetrate the deepest regions of the soul, usually because the one who gives such sermons has himself experienced pain and suffering. I have read many books of poetry, and a high percentage of them are passionless, without life or soul. This is because their authors never endured hardship, and because they were composed among surroundings of comfort. Hence the works of such authors were cold like blocks of ice. I have read books filled with sermons that do not shake a hair on the body of the listener and that lack an atom's weight of impact. The orator (whose sermons were put to print) is not speaking with feeling and sentiment, or in other words, pain and suffering. They say with their mouths, that which is not in their hearts. (Quran 3:167)

If you wish to affect and influence others, whether it is with your speech or with your poetry, or even with your actions, you must first feel the passion inside of you. You must be moved yourself by the meanings of what you are trying to convey. Then, and then only, you will come to realize that you have an influence upon others.

The blessing of knowledge

And Allah taught you that which you knew not. And Ever-Great is the Grace of Allah unto you [0 ' Muhammad]. (Quran -1:113) Ignorance kills one's conscience and soul. I admonish you, lest you be one of the ignorant. (Quran 11:46)

Knowledge is a light that leads to wisdom. It is life for one's soul and fuel for one's character. Happiness and high-spiritedness come with enlightenment, because through knowledge, one may fulfill his goals and discover what was previously hidden from him.

The soul, by its very nature longs for the acquisition of new knowledge to stimulate it and the mind. Ignorance is boredom and grief, because the ignorant person leads a life that never offers anything new or mind provoking. Yesterday is like today, which in turn is like tomorrow. If you desire happiness, then seek out knowledge and enlightenment, and you will find that anxiety, depression, and grief will leave you. If someone is ignorant, let him not be proud of either his wealth or his status in society: his life is lacking in meaning and his achievements are woefully incomplete.

The art of happiness

Among the greatest of blessings is to have a calm, stable, and happy heart. For in happiness the mind is clear, enabling one to be a productive person. It has been said that happiness is an art that needs to be learned.

And if you learn it, you will be blessed in this life. But how does one learn it? A basic principle of achieving happiness is having an ability to endure and to cope with any situation. Therefore you should neither be swayed nor governed by difficult circumstances, nor should you be annoyed by insignificant trifles. Based on the purity of the heart and its ability to endure, a person will shine. When you train yourself to be patient and forbearing, then hardship and calamity will be easy for you to bear.

The opposite of being content is being shortsighted, being concerned for no one but one's own self and forgetting about the world and all that is in it. Allah described his enemies as follows: Thinking about themselves [as how to save their own selves, ignoring the others and the Prophet]. (Quran 3:154) It is as if such people see themselves as being the whole universe or at least at the center of it. They think not of others, nor do they live for anyone but themselves.

It is incumbent upon you and me to take time out to be preoccupied with more than just us, and to sometimes distance ourselves from our own problems in order to forget our wounds and hurts. By doing this we gain two things: we make ourselves happy, and we bring joy to others. Basic to the art of happiness is to bridle our thoughts and to restrain them not allowing them to wander, stray, escape, or go wild. For if you were to leave your thoughts to wander as they wish, then they will run wild and control you. They will open the catalogue of your past woes. They will remind you of the history of your misfortunes, beginning from the day that your n1other gave you birth. If your thoughts are left to roam then they will bring to you images of past difficulties and images of a future that is frightening. These thoughts will shake your very being and will cause your feelings to flare.

Therefore bridle them, and restrain them by directing them to the concentrated application of the kind of serious thought that begets fruitful and beneficial work. Also among the principles of the art of happiness is to value life on this earth according to its true merit and worth. This life is frivolous and does not warrant anything from you except that you turn away from it. This life is filled with calamities, aches, and wounds. If that is the description of this life, then how can one be unduly affected by its minor calamities, and how can one grieve over such material things as have passed him by? The best moments of life are tainted, its future promises are mere mirages, the successful ones in it are envied, the one who is blessed is constantly threatened, and lovers are struck down by some unexpected misfortune. And in a hadith:

"Verily, knowledge is only acquired by the practice of learning, and tolerance is acquired by the practice of tolerating."

If one were to attempt to apply the meaning of this hadith to the topic under discussion, then he could go one step further and say that happiness is acquired by assuming it. It is acquired by constantly smiling, by hunting for the reasons that make one happy, and even by forcing it onto one's own self, however awkward that may seem. One does all of these things until happiness becomes second nature.

The truth of the matter is that you cannot remove from yourself all remnants of grief. This is considered to be a proof that grief will not be removed from them except in Paradise. Likewise grudges and bitterness will not be completely removed except in Paradise. And We shall remove from their breasts any sense of injury [that they may have]. (Quran 15:4 7)

So when a person knows the nature of this world and its qualities, he comes to realize that it is dry, deceitful, and unworthy; and he comes to fully understand that that is its nature and its description. An Arab poet said: "You have taken an oath not to betray us in our pacts, and it is as if you have vowed that in the end, you shall deceive us."

If the description of this world is as I have described it to be, then it is worthy of the intelligent person not to help it in its onslaught nor to surrender to depression and anxiety. What we should do is defend ourselves from all feelings that may spoil our lives, in a war that we must wage with all the strength that we have been endowed with.

The art of happiness- Pause to reflect

Do not be sad. If you are poor, then someone else is immersed in debt. If you do not own your own means of transportation, then someone else has been deprived of his legs. If you have reason to complain concerning the pains of sickness, then someone else has been bedridden for years. And if you have lost a child, then someone else has lost many children, for instance, in a single car accident. Do not be sad. You are a Muslim who believes in Allah, His Messengers, His angels, the Hereafter, and Preordainment -both the good and the bad of it. While you are blessed with this faith, which is the greatest of blessings, others disbelieve in Allah, discredit the Messengers, differ among themselves concerning the Book, deny the Hereafter, and deviate in their understanding of Divine Preordainment.

Do not be sad, because if you are, you disturb your soul and heart, and you prevent yourself from sleeping. One of the Arab poets said: "How often is that young man overcome with despair when afflicted? And with Allah is the way out, The situation becomes unbearable, and when its rope tightens, it snaps, and throughout, he never thought that he would be saved."

Controlling one's emotions

Emotions flare up for two reasons: either for joy or for inner pain. In a hadith, the Prophet (Blessings and Peace be upon him) said: "Verily, I have been prohibited from emitting two foolish and wicked sounds, one that is emitted when something favorable happens, and the other that is expressed when calamity strikes."

In order that you may not be sad over matters that you fail to get, nor rejoice because of that which has been given to you. (Quran 57:23)

For this reason, the Prophet (pbuh) said: "Verily, true patience is that which is displayed during the initial shock."

Therefore, when one contains his emotions upon both the joyful and the calamitous occasion, he is likely to achieve peace and tranquility, happiness and comfort, and the taste of triumph over his own self. Allah described man as being exultant and boastful, irritable, discontented when evil touches him, and niggardly when good touches him. The exceptions, Allah informed us, are those who remain constant in prayer. For they are on a middle path in times of both joy and sorrow. They are thankful during times of ease and are patient during times of hardship.

Unbridled emotions can greatly wear a person out, causing pain and loss of sleep. When such a person becomes angry, he flares up, threatens others, loses all self-control, and surpasses the boundaries of justice and balance. Meanwhile, if he becomes happy, he is in a state of rapture and wildness. In his intoxication of joy, he forgets himself and surpasses the bounds of modesty. When he renounces and relinquishes the company of others, he disparages them, forgetting their virtues while stamping out their good qualities. On the other hand, if he loves others, then he spares no pains in according them all forms of veneration and honor, portraying them as being the pinnacles of perfection. The Prophet (pbuh) said: "Love the one who is beloved to you in due moderation, for perhaps the day will come when you will abhor him. And hate the one whom you detest in due moderation, for perhaps the day will arrive when you will come to love him."

The bliss of the Prophet's Companions

Our Prophet Muhammad (Blessings and Peace be upon him) came to all people with a heavenly message. He was not driven by worldly ambition, he had no treasure from which to spend, no splendid gardens from which to eat, and no castle in which to live. Despite all this, his loving followers pledged allegiance to him and remained steadfast, enduring a hard life full of difficulties. They were few and weak, always in fear of being uprooted by those surrounding them, and yet they loved the Prophet (pbuh) wholly and completely. They were besieged in a mountain pass, and during that time, they had little or no food. Their reputations were attacked their own relatives waged war against them, and yet their love for him was perfect.

Some of them were dragged over the hot sands of the desert some were imprisoned, and others were subjected to inventive and innovative ways of punishment - all of which the disbelievers inflicted upon them. Having to endure all of that, they still loved him unreservedly with heart and soul. They were deprived of home, country, family, and wealth. They were driven out from the playing fields of their childhood and from the homes in which they were raised.

Despite all this suffering, they loved him unequivocally. The believers faced trials because of his message. The very ground under them was shaken violently, and yet their love for him continued to grow.

The best among their youth constantly had swords hanging menacingly over their heads. Their men moved forward lightly across the battlefield, advancing to death as if they were upon an excursion or a holiday, for the simple reason that they loved him unconditionally. One of them was charged with the duty of carrying the Prophet's message to a king in a foreign land, and that person knew that it was a mission from which he would not return. Yet he went and fulfilled his duty. One of them was sent on a mission knowing that it would be the cause of his death, and he went happily, for he loved the Prophet (pbuh) with unmitigated love. But why did they love him, and why were they so happy with his message and content with his example? Why did they forget the pain the suffering, and the hardship that resulted from following him? To put it simply he epitomized benevolence and righteousness. They perceived in him all the signs of truth and purity.

He was a symbol for those who sought out higher things. With his tenderness he cooled the rancor from the hearts of people, with words of truth he soothed their chests, and with his message he filled their souls with peace.

He poured happiness into their hearts, until the pain that they endured from being at his side was made to seem insignificant. And he instilled into their souls a belief that made them forget every injury and every adversity that they had to endure. He polished their insides with his guidance and he illuminated their eyes with his brilliance. He removed from them the burdens of ignorance the depravities of idolatry, and the evil consequences of polytheism. He extinguished the fires of malice and animosity from their souls and he poured the water of faith into their hearts. Thus, their minds and bodies became tranquil and their hearts found peace. They tasted the beauty of life with him and they knew delight in his company.

They found happiness at his side, safety and salvation in following him, and inner-richness in emulating him.

Repel boredom from your life

One who lives a life of repetition and routine will almost inevitably become a victim of boredom especially since man by his very nature tires from a lack of change. For this reason Allah, the Exalted, the Almighty, gave us variety in times and places, in food and drink - diversity in the many forms of creation: night and day, valley and mountain, white and black, hot and cold, shade and sun sweet and sour.

You should contemplate the many forms of worship that are legislated in Islam. There are deeds of the heart, of the tongue, of the limbs, and of wealth by spending it for a good cause. The prayer, alms giving, fasting, pilgrimages to Makkah fighting in the way of Allah - these are only some examples of worship.

The prayer involves standing, bowing, prostrating, and sitting. If you desire relaxation, vitality, and continued productivity, then bring diversity into your work, your reading, and your daily life. In terms of reading for example, read a broad range of topics: the Quran its explanation the biography of the Prophet (Blessings and Peace be upon him) and his Companions, hadith.

Islamic jurisprudence, history, literature, books of general knowledge, and so forth. Distribute your time between worship and enjoying what is lawful, from visiting friends, entertaining guests, playing sports, or going on excursions: you will find yourself to be a lively and bright person, because the soul delights in variety and things that are new.

Cast off anxiety

Do not be sad, for your Lord says: Have We not opened your breast for you [O'Muhammad]? (Quran 94:1)

The message of this verse embraces all those who carry the truth, who see the light, and who tread the path of guidance.

Is he whose breast Allah has opened to Islam, so that he is in light from His Lord [as he who is non-Muslim]? So, woe to those whose hearts are hardened against the remembrance of Allah! (Quran 39:22)

Therefore there is a truth that causes the heart to be opened and a falsehood that causes it to harden, and whosoever Allah wills to guide, He opens his breast to Islam. (Quran 6:125)

So the acceptance of and adherence to this Religion is a goal that cannot be achieved except by the one who is blessed.

'Be not sad [or afraid] surely Allah is with us. (Quran 9:40)

Do not be sad: live today as if it were the last day of your life. With this frame of mind and outlook towards life, you have no reason to allow sadness or anger to steal the little time you have. In a hadith the Prophet (Blessings and Peace be upon him) said:

"When the morning comes upon you, then do not expect to see the evening, and when you see the night, do not expect to see the morning."

In other words, live with heart, body, and soul for today only, without dwelling upon the past and without being anxious about the future. An Arab poet said:

"The past is lost forever, and that which is hoped for is from the unseen, so all that you have is the present hour."

Being preoccupied with the past and dragging past woes into the present - these are the signs of an unstable and unsound mind. A Chinese proverb reads: "Do not cross the bridge until you reach it." In other words, be anxious over events only when they come to pass. One of our pious predecessors said, "O' son of Adam, verily, you have only three days: Yesterday, and it has forsaken you; tomorrow, and it has yet to arrive; and today, so fear Allah and obey Him in it." How can he truly live who carries with him the concerns of the past, the present, and the future? How can one find peace, while constantly recollecting that which has already occurred? One plays a past event back in his mind feels its pain, and yet benefits nothing from the process. The meaning of, 'when the morning comes, do not expect to see the evening, and when the evening comes, do not expect to see the morning,' is that we should not have lofty or long-term hopes for this world.

Expect death and do your best in doing good deeds. Do not let your concerns and ambitions surpass the limit of that day in which you live, a code that will allow you to concentrate and spend all of your energies on being productive each day. Use time efficiently and concentrate all of your efforts on achieving something today, by improving your manners, taking care of your health, and improving your relations with others.

Cast off anxiety - Pause to reflect

Do not be sad, for that which has been preordained has already been decided upon and will take place though you may not like it. The pens have dried, the scrolls have been rolled up, and every affair is firmly established. Therefore your sadness will not change your reality in the least.

Do not be sad, because, with your sadness, you desire for time's suspension: for the sun to stop in its place, for the hands of the clock to stand still, for the steps of your feet to move backwards, and for the river to flow back to its source.

Do not be sad, because sadness is like a hurricane that violently tosses the waves, changing the atmosphere and destroying the blooming flowers of the luxuriant garden.

Do not be sad, because the one who is sad is like a person who pours water into a bucket that has a hole in it. He is like a writer who uses his finger to write on water.

Do not be sad, because the true span of life is measured by the number of days in which you are content.

Do not then spend your days in grief, do not waste your nights in sorrow, and do not be extravagant in squandering your time; for truly, Allah loves not those who are extravagant and wasteful. Do not be sad, for in truth, your Lord forgives sins and accepts repentance. His mercy and forgiveness for those who believe in the Trinity - that is, if they repent: In an authentic hadith the Prophet (pbuh) said: "Allah, blessed is He and Most High, says: 'O' son of Adam, indeed you will not supplicate to Me and hope from Me except that I will forgive you, in proportion to what came from you (i.e. your level of sincerity), and I won't mind. O' son of Adam, if your sins were to reach in magnitude the height of the heavens, and then you were to ask Me for forgiveness, I would forgive you, and I won't mind. O' son of Adam, were you to come to Me with sins that (in their size) almost fill the earth, and you met Me without ascribing to Me any partners, I would come to you with its size in forgiveness."

Bukhari related that the Prophet (pbuh) said: "Indeed, Allah extends His Hand in the night to forgive the one who sins in the day, and He extends His Hand in the day to forgive the one who sins at night, and this continues until the sun rises from the west."

In another hadith, the Prophet (pbuh) relates that Allah said: "O' my slaves, verily you sin by day and night, and I forgive all sins; so seek forgiveness from Me and I will forgive you."

In another authentic hadith, the Prophet (pbuh) said: "By the One Who has my soul in His Hand, if you were not to sin, then Allah would remove you, and would bring another nation who sins, and who then seek forgiveness from Allah; and He would forgive them." And the Prophet (Blessings and Peace be upon him) also said: "By the One Who has my soul in His Hand, if you were not to sin, then I would fear upon you that which is more severe than sin; and that is self-conceit."

In another authentic narration, the Prophet (pbuh) said: "Every one of you is constantly doing wrong, and the best of those who constantly do wrong are the ones who are constantly making repentance."

He (pbuh) also said in this authentic hadith: "Truly, Allah is happier with the repentance of His slave than one of you who is on his mount, and upon his mount is his drink and food; then he loses his mount in the desert, and he searches for it until he loses hope; so he sleeps and then wakes up to find that his mount is beside him, and he says, 'O' Allah, you are my slave and I am your Lord'. He pronounced this mistake as a result of his extreme happiness."

He (pbuh) is also authentically reported to have said: "Verily, a slave (of Allah) commits a sin and then he says, 'O' Allah, forgive me my sin, for indeed, none forgives sins except You.

Then he commits another sin, and he afterwards says, O' Allah forgive me my sin, for indeed, none forgives sins except You'. Then he commits another sin, and he afterwards says, O' Allah, forgive me my sin, for indeed none forgives sins except You . Then Allah says, My slave knows that he has a Lord, Who takes one to account for sins, and Who also forgives sins, so let my slave do as he wishes." The meaning of this is that as long as Allah's servants is contrite and repentant, then Allah will forgive him.

Do not be sad - Everything twill occur according to pre-ordainment

Everything occurs according to preordainment and according to what has been decreed. Such is the belief of Muslims, the followers of Muhammad (Blessings and Peace be upon him). And nothing happens in the Universe except through Allah's Knowledge. Permission, and Divine Plan.

In a hadith the Prophet (pbuh) said: "Wonderful is the affair of the believer! His affairs in their entirety are good for him: if good befalls him he is thankful, and that is good for him. And if harm befalls him, he is patient, and that is good for him. And this (prosperous state of being) is only for the believer."

In an authentic hadith, the Prophet (pbuh) said: "If you ask, then ask of Allah, and if you seek help then seek it from Allah. And know that if the whole of the nation were to rally together in order to bring benefit to you in anything, they would not benefit you except with that which Allah has written for you. And if they were to gather together in order to inflict harm upon you with something, they would not harm you except with that which Allah has written upon you. The pens have been raised and the pages have dried."

The Prophet (Blessings and Peace be upon him) also said: "And know that what has befallen you was not going to miss you, and that which missed you was not meant to befall you."

In another authentic hadith, the Prophet (pbuh) said: "Strive for that which will benefit you, seek help from Allah, do not be weak, and do not say: If I had done such and such, the situation would be such and such. But say: Allah has decreed and what He wishes, He does."

And in another authentic hadith, the Prophet (pbuh) said: "Every matter that Allah decrees for His slave is better for him."

Do not be sad - Wait patiently for ta happy outcome

The following hadith is found in the book of At-Tirmidhi: "The best form of worship is to wait (patiently) for a happy outcome."

The morning of the afflicted is looming, so watch for it. An Arab proverb says, "If the rope becomes too tight, it will snap."

In other words, if a situation reaches the level of crisis, then expect a light and an opening to appear. Allah says: And whosoever fears Allah and keeps his duty to Him, He will remit his sins from him, and will enlarge his reward. (Quran 65:5) And whosoever fears Allah and keeps his duty to Him, He will make his matter easy for him. (Quran 65:4)

In an authentic hadith, the Prophet (Blessings and Peace be upon him) relates this saying from Allah: "I am with the thoughts of My slave towards Me, so let him think of Me as he pleases."

As carrying the burdens of anxiety is madness. There is your Lord, who provided you with solutions to yesterday, And He will similarly provide for what is to come tomorrow."

'Let events flow in their predestined path, And do not sleep except with a clear mind, Between the period of the blinking of the eye and its opening, Allah changes things from one state to another.

Wait patiently for ta happy outcome - Pause to reflect

Do not worry about your wealth that is stored in vaults. Unless you have faith in Allah, your high castles and your green gardens will only bring you worry, grief, and hopelessness. Do not be sad: even the diagnosis of the doctor and his medicine cannot make you happy if you have allowed sadness to dwell in your heart, letting it permeate your emotions and your existence. Do not be sad: you have the ability to supplicate to Allah and thus excel at humbling yourself at the doorstep of the King of kings. You have the blessed last third of the night to invoke Allah and to rub your head upon the ground in prostration.

Do not be sad: Allah has created for you the earth and what is in it. He has caused gardens of beauty to grow, filling them with many kinds of plants and flowers in pairs, both male and female. And He has made tall palm trees, shining stars, forests, rivers and streams - yet you are sad! Do not be sad: you drink water that is pure, you breathe fresh air, you walk upon your two feet in health, and you sleep the evenings in peace. Do not be sad: Seek forgiveness from Allah often, for your Lord is Oft-Forgiving.

The Prophet (Blessings and Peace be upon him) said: "Whosoever seeks forgiveness (from Allah) often, then Allah makes for him a good ending for every matter of concern and provides for him a way out of every tight situation."

Do not be sad - Always Remember Allah

Concerning His remembrance, Allah, the All-Glorious, says: Verily, in the remembrance of Allah do hearts find rest. The Prophet (Blessings and Peace be upon him) also said: "Shall I not inform you of the best of deeds, and the purest of them with your Lord? The deed which is better for you than spending gold and silver (for a good cause), and which is better for you than to meet your enemy, and you cut their throats and they cut yours?" They said, "Yes_ O' Messenger of Allah." He said, "The remembrance of Allah."

The following is an authentic hadith: "A man came to the Prophet and said, 'O' Messenger of Allah, the com1nandments of Islam have become too much or me, and I am old in age; so inform of something that I can adhere to.' He said, 'That your tongue (continually) remains moist with the remembrance of Allah.'"

Do not be sad - Never lose hope of Allah's mercy

Certainly no one despairs of Allah's Mercy, except the people who disbelieve. (Quran 12:87)

Do not grieve over the hurt that is inflicted upon you by others, and forgive those that have ill-treated you. The price of jealousy and rancor is enormous it is the price that the revengeful person pays in exchange for his malice towards others. He pays with his heart flesh, and blood. His peace, his relaxation, and his happiness - these he forsakes because he desires the sweetness of revenge and because he resent s others. Jealousy and rancor are illnesses for which Allah has given the cure and remedy.

[Those] who repress anger, and who pardon men. (Quran 3:134)

Show forgiveness, enjoin what is good, and turn away from the foolish [i.e. don't punish them]. (Quran 7:199)

Repel [the evil] with one which is better [i.e. Allah ordered the faithful believers to be patient at the time of anger, and to excuse those who treat them badly] then verily.' He, between whom and you there was enmity, [will become] as though he was a close friend. (Quran 41:34)

Do not grieve over that which has passed you by in life, for indeed you have been blessed with much.

Contemplate the many favors and gifts that Allah has bestowed upon you and be thankful to Him for them. Remind yourself of Allah's many blessings for He, the Almighty, said:

And if you would count the graces of Allah, never could you be able to count them. (Quran 16:18)

And [Allah] has completed and perfected His Graces upon you, [both] apparent [i.e. Islamic Monotheism, and the lawful pleasures of this world, including health, good looks, etc.] and hidden [i.e. One's Faith in Allah (of Islamic Monotheism) knowledge, wisdom, guidance for doing righteous deeds, and also the pleasures and delights of the Hereafter in Paradise, etc.]. (Quran 31:20) And whatever of blessings and good things you have, it is from Allah. Then, when harm touches you, unto Him you cry aloud for help. (Quran 16:53)

Allah said, establishing His favors upon man: Have We not made for him a pair of eyes; and a tongue and a pair of lips? And shown him the two ways [good and evil]? (Quran 90: 8-10)

Life, health the faculties of hearing and seeing, two hands and two legs, water, air, food - these are some of the more visible blessings in this world while the greatest of all blessings is that of Islam and correct guidance. What would you say to someone who offered you large sums of money in return for your eyes, your ears, your legs, your hands or your heart?

How great is your wealth in reality? By not being thankful you do not render justice to Allah's countless favors.

Grieve not over unworthy things

By being unconcerned over trifles, you display a virtue that will bring you happiness, for the one who is lofty in his aims is engrossed only with concern for the Hereafter. One of our pious predecessors advised one of his brothers with the following words, "Be concerned about this only: about meeting Allah, about standing in front of Him, and about the Hereafter."

That Day shall you be brought to Judgment, not a secret of you will be hidden. (Quran 69:18)

There is not a single worry or concern whose significance is not diminished when it is compared to the concerns of the Hereafter. What are the worries of this life? They are status, prestige, fame, income, wealth, mansions, and children. They are all nothing when compared to the accountability before Allah!

Allah described His enemies, the hypocrites, by saying: While another party was thinking about themselves [as how to save their own selves, ignoring the others and the Prophet] and thought wrongly of Allah. (Quran 3:154)

Their concerns are for themselves their stomachs, and their lusts; they know nothing of higher motives. When the people pledged allegiance to the Prophet (pbuh) under the tree, one of the hypocrites left hastily in search of his red camel, which had strayed. He said, "For me to find my camel is more beloved to me than your ceremony of pledging allegiance." And in relation to this incident, the following is related in a hadith: "All of you have been forgiven, except for the owner of the red camel."

One of the hypocrites, who was worried only about himself, said to his companions concerning the expedition to Tabuk, "March not forth in the heat." Allah, the Exalted, said: Say: 'The Fire of Hell is more intense in heat'. (Quran 9:81)

Another one of them said: 'Grant me leave [to be exempted from Jihad] and put me not into trial. · (Quran 9:49)

And Allah said: Surely, they have fallen into trial. (Quran 9:49)

While yet others were troubled and concerned only for their wealth and their families: 'Our possessions and our families occupied us, so ask forgiveness for us. (Quran 48:11)

These concerns are trifles that none should be preoccupied with except for those who are themselves trifling and insignificant. As for the noble Companions they desired the favors of Allah and they longed for His pleasure.

Do not be sad - Repel anxiety

Idleness is destructive, and most people who suffer from worries and anxieties are the same people who are idle and inactive. Rumors and gossip are the only dividends for those that are bankrupt of meaningful and fruitful work. Apply yourself to something and work hard at it. Read, recite, and glorify your Lord with praises. Write, visit friends, and benefit from your time. In short, do not give a single minute away to idleness. The day that you do will be the day that anxieties and worries will find their way into your life. Superstition and evil whispers will enter your mind, allowing you to become a playground for the games of the devil.

Do not grieve over the person who forgets or denies the favors you once gave to him for your desire should be solely for the reward of Allah.

Perform righteous deeds purely and sincerely for the pleasure of Allah, and do not expect either congratulation or gratitude from any person. Do not take it to heart if you confer a favor upon someone and he then turns out to be ungrateful showing no sign of appreciation for what you have done. Seek your reward from Allah. Allah says of His righteous slaves:

They seek Bounties from Allah and His pleasure. (Quran 59:8)

Say: 'No reward do I ask of you for this' (Quran 25:57)

So make your dealings with Allah alone, as He is the One Who rewards people for good deeds. He gives and He bestows or He punishes and He takes to account, being pleased with those who do well and angry with those who do evil. Martyrs were killed in Qandahar, and 'Umar (may Allah be pleased with him) asked the companions. "Who was killed?"

They mentioned some names to him, and then they said, "And people whom you do not know." 'Umar's eyes filled with tears and he said, "But Allah knows them."

A pious person fed the best and finest of food to a blind man. His family said to him, "This blind man does not know what he is eating (so give him something of lower quality)." He replied. "But Allah knows!"

Since Allah knows your deeds, knows of the good you do and the help you give to others, remain carefree and untroubled about what people think.

Grieve not when others blame and disparage you

A poet said: "The vast ocean feels no harm, when the boy pitches into it a rock."

Grieve not over being poor

The more the body enjoys, the more the soul become sullied, and there is safety in having little. Taking only that which you need from this world is an early comfort that Allah bestows upon those whom He pleases among His slaves.

Verily! We will inherit the earth and whatsoever is thereon. (Quran 19:40)

One poet said: "Water, bread, and shade, these form a most worthy bliss, I have denied the favors of my Lord, if I said that I had too little."

What in this world is truly important, but cold water, warm bread, and plentiful shade!

Do not feel sad over fears for what may happen

In the Torah, the following has been related: "Most of what is feared to occur, never happens!"

This means that most apprehensions and fears of impending difficulty fail to take shape in reality. Conjectures of the mind are far greater in number and in scope than the things that actually happen in life. An Arab poet said: "I said to my heart when it was attacked by a fit of anxiety, be happy, because most fears are false." This implies that if you hear of an impending calamity, or hear of oncoming disaster, don't be overly alarmed, especially since the majority of predictions about impending harm are false.

Grieve not over criticism from the jealous and the weak-minded

You will be rewarded if you show forbearance to their criticism and to their impertinent remarks. The more they criticize you, the more you are increased in worth, because only someone who is unaccomplished has no one who is jealous of him, and according to the Arab saying, "People do not kick a dead dog."

One poet said: "They are jealous of he who has surpassed them, People show him enmity and opposition. Just like spiteful women, who speak of the fair maiden. With jealousy and malice -that she is of a low and base character." Zuhayr said: "They are jealous of that which he has been blessed with, Allah will not take away from him the cause of their resentment." Another said: "They will envy my death, what wretchedness is this, Even in my death, I am not spared from their jealousy." In another poem: "If a person reaches the sky with his nobleness, then his enemies will be the numbers of the stars in the sky, They shoot at him using a bow with every kind of persecution, Yet their abuses will never bring them to the level of his nobility." Prophet Musa (Moses) asked his Lord to prevent people from abusing him with their tongues. Allah said, "O' Musa, I have not done so for myself. I have created them and provided for them and they blaspheme and curse me!"

It has been authentically narrated that the Prophet (Blessings and Peace be upon him) said, "Allah says: 'The son of Adam curses Me and blasphemes Me, and he has no right to do so. As for his cursing Me, he curses the time, and I am the time: I alternate the day and night as I please. As for their blaspheming Me, they say that I have a wife and a child, and I have neither a wife nor a child.'"

You may not be able to prevent people from attacking your honor, but you are able to do well, and ultimately, to ignore and turn away from their criticism and scorn.

Another poet said: "I move past the fool who curses me, and I continue on my previous course saying: he does not refer to me!"

And yet another said: "When the fool speaks, then do not respond to him, for better than to answer him is silence."

Idiots and fools clearly feel insulted by those who shine, those who are noble, and those who display genius.

"If the strengths and good points that I possess, were my sins, then pray tell me, how can I make amends?" Woe to every slanderer and backbite1 Who has gathered wealth and counted it. He thinks that this wealth will make him last forever! Nay! Verily, he will be thrown into the crushing Fire. (Quran 104:1-4) A well-known western writer said, "Do what is right, and then tum your back to every vulgar criticism."

Do not respond to an injurious statement that is made about you.

Forbearance buries faults, tolerance is superior silence conquers the enemy, and forgiveness is honor for which you shall be rewarded. If defamatory remarks are printed about you know that half of those that read such things quickly forget them while the other half are uninterested in the first place.

So do not create further noise and fuss by refuting what has been said. A wise person said: "People are oblivious of you and me, and are busily striving for their bread. And if one of them is thirsty, he will forget my death and yours."

A poet said: Do not broadcast your affairs to your sitting companions. Because they are jealous and will rejoice at your misfortune." A house that has within it serenity and bread is better than a house that is replete with many kinds of expensive foods, yet is a place of trouble and unrest.

Stop to reflect

Do not be sad: for sickness is a transient state of being; the sin can be forgiven; the debt will be repaid; the captive will be released; the beloved one who is abroad will return ; the sinner will repent ; and the poor will be increased in their wealth.

Do not be sad, for do you not see how the black clouds disperse and the violent winds subside? Your hardships will be followed by comfort and your future is bright.

Do not be sad, for the blaze of the sun is extinguished by luxuriant shade; the thirst of noon is refreshed by fresh water; the pangs of hunger find relief in bread; and the anxiety of sleeplessness is followed by calm repose ; the pains of sickness are soon forgotten after the return of health. It is only upon you to forbear for a short time and to be patient for a few moments.

Do not be sad, for even doctors, wise men, scholars, and poets are weak and unable to defy or change that which has been decreed. D not despair when you meet with affliction that weakens your spirit, since the closest one comes to relief, is when he loses all hope.

Do not be sad: select for yourself that which Allah has chosen for you.

Stand if He causes you to stand and sit if He orders you to sit. Show patience if He has made you to be poor and be thankful if He makes you to be rich. These points are understood from the statement, "I am pleased with Allah as my Lord with Islam as a Religion, and with Muhammad as a Messenger."

And an Arab poet said: "Do not weave a plan for yourself, the people of plotting are destroyed, be contented with our decree, We are worthier to plan for you than you yourself."

Do not be sad: overlook the actions of others. They can lay no claim on giving benefit or harm death or life, reward or punishment. We live such a life (of amazing pleasure in the worship of Allah) that if the kings knew about it, they would fight us over it with swords.

The heart sometimes dances rapturously, from the happiness of remembering Allah and of feeling close to Him." A wise person once said: What can my enemies do to me! My garden and my paradise are in my breast, wherever I go they are with me. If my enemies kill me, I become a martyr and if they banish me from my country, I go abroad as a tourist; and by imprisoning me, they allow me to have solitude (so that I can worship Allah). What has he found who has lost Allah, and what has he discovered who has found Allah? They can never be equal; the one who has found Allah has found everything and the one who has lost Him has lost everything. Do not blindly feel grief; instead, make sure you know the value of the thing over which you feel sad. The Prophet (Peace be upon him) said: "For me to say, 'How perfect is Allah, All praise is for Him, there is none worthy of worship except Him, and Allah is the greatest,' is more beloved to me than all that the sun rises upon."

Of rich people their castles, houses, and wealth, one of our pious predecessors said: "We eat and they eat. We drink and they drink. We see and they see. We will not be called to account and they will be held accountable (i.e. for their wealth, how it was acquired and how it was spent).

In the words of a poet: "The first night in the grave causes one to forget, the castles of Khosrau and the treasures of Caesar."

Allah said: And truly you have come unto Us alone without wealth, companions or anything else, as We created you the first time. (Quran 6:94)

The believers say: This is what Allah and His Messenger [Muhammad] had promised us, and Allah and His Messenger had spoken the truth. (Quran 33:22)

And the hypocrites say: Allah and his Messenger promised us nothing but delusions! (Quran 33:12) Your life is the product of your thoughts.

The thoughts that you invest in will have an indelible effect upon your life, regardless of whether they are happy thoughts or miserable thoughts.

A poet said: "Fear does not fill my heart before the occurrence of that which is feared, and I don't become overly distressed if that event does occur."

Do not be sad - Do good to others

Being of service to others leads to happiness. In an authentic hadith the Prophet (Blessings and Peace be upon him) said: "Verily, Allah will say to His slave as He is taking account of him on the Day of Judgment. 'O' son of Adam, I was hungry and you did not feed Me.' He will answer, 'How can I feed You and You are the Lord of the worlds!' He will say, 'Did you not know that My slave so and so who is the son of so and so felt hunger, and you did not feed him. Alas! Had you fed him you would have found that (i.e. reward) with Me.

O' son of Adam, I was thirsty and you gave Me nothing to drink.' He will say, 'How can I give You drink, and You are the Lord of the worlds!' He will say, 'Did you not know that My slave so and so, the son of so and so felt thirsty and you did not give him drink. Alas! If you had given him, you would have found that (i.e. reward) with Me. O' son of Adam, I became sick and you did not visit Me.' He will say, 'How can I visit You and You are the Lord of the worlds!' He will say, 'Did you not know that My slave so and so, the son of so and so became sick and you did not visit him. Alas! Had you visited him, you would have found Me with him.'"

Here is an interesting point; in the last third of the hadith are the words: "...you would have found Me with him."

This is unlike the first two parts of the hadith: "You would have found that (i.e. the reward for feeding and giving drink) with Me."

The reason for the difference is that Allah, the All-Merciful is with those whose hearts are troubled as is the case with the person who is sick. And in another hadith, the Prophet (pbuh) said: "There is reward in each moist liver (i.e. to do service to any living creature will be rewarded)."

Also, know that Allah admitted the prostitute from the children of Israel into Paradise because she gave a drink to a dog that was thirsty. So what will be the case for the one who feeds other humans, giving them drink and removing from them hardships!

In an authentic hadith, the Prophet (pbuh) said, "Whoever has extra provision should give from it to the one who has no provision. And whoever has an extra mount should give with this extra to the one who has no mount."

Ibn Mubarak's neighbor was a Jew. He would always feed him before feeding his own children and would provide clothing for him first and then for his children. Some people said to the Jew, "Sell us your house." He answered, "My house is for two thousand dinars. One thousand is for the price of the house and one thousand is for having my friend as a neighbor! Ibn Mubarak heard of this and he exclaimed." O'Allah, guide him to Islam." Then, by the permission of Allah he accepted Islam.

On another occasion. Ibn Mubarak passed by a caravan of people who were traveling to make the pilgrimage to Makkah, and he too was on his way to do the same. He saw one of the women from the caravan take a dead crow from a cesspit. He sent his servant to inquire about this and when he asked her, she replied. "We have had nothing for three days except that which finds its way into it." When Ibn Mubarak heard of this, his eyes swelled with tears.

He ordered for all of his provision to be distributed among those of the caravan, and having nothing with which to continue the journey he returned to his home and gave up making the pilgrimage e for that year. Later, he saw someone in a dream saying, "Your pilgrimage has been accepted, as have your rites; and your sins have been forgiven."

Allah says: And give them preference over themselves, even though they were in need of that themselves)

(Quran 59:9)

One poet said: "Even if I am a person who is far, From his friend in terms of distance, I offer him my help and wish to alleviate his difficulties, And I answer his invitation and his call to me for help, And if he dons a wonderful new outfit I will not say, Alas, were I to be blessed with the clothes that he wears."

By Allah, how wonderful are good manners and a generous soul! No one regrets having done well even if he was extravagant in doing so. Regret is only for the mistake or for the wrong done, even when that wrong is a minor one.

Jealousy is not something new

If you hear the beating of resentful words in your ears, do not worry -jealousy is not something new. As a poet said: "Devote yourself to the gathering of virtues, and work, And tum your back on someone who cools his jealousy by givmg you censure, Know that your life's-span is the season of good deeds, In it, they may be accepted, and after his death, when all jealousy ceases."

A wise person said: "When facing criticism or the unjust rebuke, those who have sensitive feelings must pour a certain amount of coolness into their nerves by force."

Another said: "The coward dies many deaths and the brave man dies one."

Ali (may Allah be pleased with him) said: "Which of the two days of death do I fear? The day in which it was not decreed for me to die or the day in which death was preordained for me. As for the former, I fear it not. And as for the latter, it is destined to happen, and even cautious ones cannot be saved on that day."

Abu Bakr (may Allah be pleased with him) said: "Seek out death (i.e. be brave) and you shall be granted life."

Stop to reflect

Do not be sad, for Allah defends you and the angels ask forgiveness for you; the believers share with you their supplications in every prayer; the Prophet (Blessings and Peace be upon him) will intercede for the believers; the Quran is replete with good promises; and above all is the mercy of He Who is the Most Merciful.

Do not be sad: the good deed is increased so that its value is multiplied tenfold or seven hundred fold or even much more.

Meanwhile, the evil deed is valued without increase or multiplication, and your Lord can forgive even that. How many times do we witness Allah's generosity, generosity that is unmatched by any! And benevolence from anyone else cannot reach even near His Benevolence. If you do not associate partners with Allah, if you believe in the true religion, and if you love Allah and His Messenger (pbuh), do not feel sad. If you feel regret for your bad deeds and you rejoice when you do a worthy act, do not feel sad. You have much good with you that you do not perceive.

If, in your life, you are able to establish the state of balanced harmony that is referred to in the following hadith, do not feel sad: "How wonderful is the state of the believer.

All of his affairs are good for him! And that is not so, except for the believer. If he has cause to be happy, he is thankful, and that is good for him. And if he is afflicted with hardship, he is patient, and that is good for him."

Do not be sad: forbearance in times of distress is the path to both success and happiness.

And endure you patiently, your patience is not but from Allah. (Quran 16:12 7)

Through patience we achieve a good life. For the people of the Sunnah, there are three things that they resort to when faced with calamity: patience supplication, and waiting with expectation for a good outcome.

A poet said: "We have poured them a glass and they have similarly poured one for us (alluding to the blood enemies draw from each other in battle), But in the face of death, we were the more patient."

The Prophet (pbuh) said: "May Allah have mercy on Musa (Moses) He was tested with more than this (i.e. than what I have been tested with), and he was still patient."

And he (pbuh) said: "Whoever is patient, Allah will give him further strength to continue to be patient."

A poet said: "I have crawled my way to distinction, and those who have striven have reached it, with the toil of labor, and the sparing of no small effort, many have tried to reach it, and most became bored or tired during their journey. And they embrace distinction that remain true and are patient. Do not consider distinction to be an apple that you eat, you will not achieve distinction until you beat hardship with your patience."

Higher goals are not achieved through dreaming or fantasizing; they can only be reached through dedication and commitment.

Do not grieve over how people treat you. And learn this lesson by observing how they behave with Allah.

Imam Ahmad reported a hadith in the book of Zuhd, in which the Prophet (pbuh) relates the following saying from Allah: "Strange are you, O' son of Adam! I have created you and you worship other than Me. I have provided for you and you thank those besides me. I show you love by giving you blessings and I do not need you. While you show me animosity through your sins and you are to me poor. My good is descending to you and your evil is rising to Me.'·

It is mentioned in the biography of Prophet Eesa (Jesus) (may peace be upon him) that, by the permission of Allah, he healed thirty sick people and cured many who were afflicted with blindness. Afterwards they turned on him as enemies.

Do not be sad from the want of ample provision

Verily, the One Who provides sustenance is Allah. He has made it binding upon Himself that whatever provision He has written for His slaves will reach them. And in the heaven is your provision, and that which you are promised. (Quran 51:22). If Allah is the One Who provides for the creation why curry favor with people? And why should one degrade himself in front of another person in the hope of procuring from him his sustenance? Allah said: And no [moving] living creature is there on earth but its provision is due from Allah. (Quran 11:6)

Whatever of mercy [i.e. [good], Allah may grant to mankind, none can withhold it, and whatever He may withhold, none can grant it thereafter) (Quran 35:2)

Do not be sad, for there are means of making it easier to bear calamity. Among them are the following:

1. Expecting reward and recompense from Allah the Exalted: Only those who are patient shall receive their rewards in full without reckoning. (Quran 39:10)

2. Visiting those who are afflicted and seeking comfort in that you are better off than many others.

A poet said: "If not for the many mourners around me, who weep for their brothers, I would have taken my own life."

So look at those who surround you. There will not be one, except that hardship or affliction has touched him. Appreciate that, compared to others, your trial is light.

If you know that your trial is not in your religion, but is in worldly matters then be content.

Know that no trick or artifice can be used to undo what has already taken place. A poet said:

"Do not use trickery to change the circumstance.

For the only trick is in leaving all trickery."

Appreciate that the choice of what is good for you or not good for you belongs only with Allah: ...and it may be that you dislike a thing which is good for you. (Quran 2:216)

Do not mimic the personality of others

For every nation there is a direction to which they face. So hasten towards all that is good. Every person has his own set of talents, abilities, skills, and preferences. One aspect of the Prophet's character was his ability to lead: he employed his Companions each in accordance with his talent and expertise. 'Ali was both just and wise, so the Prophet (Blessings and Peace be upon him) appointed him to be a judge.

To melt into the personality of another, for whatever reason is akin to suicide. And to imitate the natural traits of others is to deliver a deathblow to one's own self. Among Allah's signs that one should marvel at are the diverse characteristics of people -such as their talents, the different languages they speak, and their different colors. Abu Bakr (may Allah be pleased with him), for example, through his gentleness and tenderness, greatly benefited Islam and this Nation. 'Umar, on the other hand, helped Islam and its adherents to be victorious through his stern demeanor and austerity. Therefore be comfortable with your inherent talents and abilities. Develop them expand on them, and benefit from them.

I have not seen or heard of anything that brings repose, honor, and dignity as much as seclusion does. It helps one to stay away from evil, it protects one's honor, and it saves time. It keeps one away from the jealous minded and those who take pleasure in your affliction.

It promotes the remembrance of the Hereafter, and it allows one to reflect on the meeting with Allah. In times of seclusion, one's thoughts may roam in that which is beneficial, in that which contains wisdom.

Only Allah knows the full benefits of seclusion, for in seclusion, one's mind develops, views are ripened, the heart finds repose, and one finds himself to be in an ideal atmosphere for worship. By remaining isolated at times one distances himself from trials, from flattering the person who deserves no praise, and from the eyes of jealous and envious persons. One is saved from the haughtiness of the proud and the follies of the idiot. In isolation one's faults, deeds, and sayings are all secluded behind a veil. During periods of isolation, one is able to delve deep into a sea of ideas and concepts. In such a state, the mind is free to form its opinions.

Isolated from the company of others, the soul is free to achieve a state of rapture and to hunt for the stimulating thought. When alone, one does nothing for show or ostentation since none but Allah sees him, and since none but Allah hears him. Every person who was a genius, a mental giant, or a great contributor to the human race watered the seeds of his greatness from the well of isolation, until the seed become a plant, and then finally, a formidable tree.

'Ali ibn 'Abdul 'Aziz said: "I never tasted the sweetness of life until I became a companion of home and book. There is nothing more honorable than knowledge, So I seek in no other an associate, Truly, the only degradation is in mixing with people, Therefore leave them and live nobly and stately."

Another said: "I found company in my solitude and I remained fervently in my home, so felicity was perpetual for me and my happiness grew, I have severed human relations and I couldn't care, whether the arn1y has gone forth or the president has given us a visit!"

A poet said, "Meeting with people brings about no benefit. So spend less time in conversing with others, though barring, the acquirement of knowledge or the improvement of one's condition."

Ibn Faris said: "They asked how I was, and I said, well, and thank you, a need is fulfilled and another is neglected. When distress is such that my heart becomes constricted, I say that perhaps one day will bring with it some aid. My comrade is my cat and my soul's companions are my books, and the object of my love is my night-lantern."

Do not be shaken by hardships

Hardship strengthens your heart, atones for your sins, and helps to suppress an inclination towards pride and haughtiness. You might remember that in times of hardship you abandoned senseless folly and you remembered Allah. When you were afflicted others extended brotherly compassion to you, and you became the fortunate recipient of the supplications of the righteous. At such times, you willfully and humbly surrendered yourself to Allah's will and resigned yourself to His decree. Affliction begets circumspection and provides the afflicted with an early warning against following the path of evil. The one upon whom calamity has fallen can display courage with patience; and his circumstances, unlike the one who is drunk with worldly pleasures permit him to solemnly prepare for a meeting with his Lord.

He is able to pass judgment on this world with an impartial ruling, and thus he will come to know it as something that is not worth pining for. Other points associated with the wisdom and benefits of sometimes facing hardship, though they might escape our comprehension, are definitely present and known to the Lord of all that exists.

Pause to think about hardships

Do not be sad, for sadness will weaken your determination and the quality of your worship. One of the offshoots of depression is that it often causes one to be pessimistic, to find blame in everyone, including - and we seek refuge in Allah - Allah Himself. Do not be sad, for sadness, grief, and anxiety are the roots of mental problems, the sources of stress. Do not be sad, for you have with you the Quran, supplication remembrance, and prayer.

You can lighten the load of your anxiety by giving others, doing well, and being productive.

Do not be sad, and do not surrender to sadness by taking the easy path of idleness and inactivity, but pray, glorify your Lord read write, work, visit relatives and friends, and reflect.

Invoke Me and ask me for anything, I will respond to your [invocation]. (Quran 40: 60)

Invoke your Lord with humility and in secret. He likes not the aggressors. (Quran 7:55)

So, call you [o ' Muhammad and the believers] upon [or invoke]

Allah making [your] worship pure for Him [Alone] [by worshipping none but Him and by doing religious deeds sincerely for Allah's sake only and not to show off and not to set up rivals with Him in Worship]. (Quran 40: 14)

Say [O' Muhammad]: 'Invoke Allah or invoke the Most Beneficent [Allah], by whatever name you invoke Him [it is the same], for to Him belong the Best Names.

Do not be sad - The fundamentals of happiness

1. Know that if you do not live within the scope of today, your thoughts will be scattered, your affairs will become confused, and your worrying will increase - these realities explain the hadith: "When you are in the morning, do not expect to see the evening, and when you are in the evening, do not expect to see the morning."

2. Forget the past and all that it contained. Being absorbed in things that are gone is sheer lunacy.

3. Do not be preoccupied with the future. Because the future is in the world of the unseen, do not let it bother you until it comes.

4. Do not be shaken by criticism, know that, in proportion to your worth, the level of people's criticism rises.

5. Faith in Allah and good deeds: these are the ingredients that make up a good and happy life.

6. Whoever desires peace, tranquility, and comfort can find it all in the remembrance of Allah.

7. You should know with certainty that everything that happens, occurs in accordance with a divine decree.

8. Do not expect gratitude from anyone.

9. Train yourself to be ready and prepared for the worst eventuality.

10. Perhaps what has happened is in your best interest (though you may not comprehend how that is so).

11. Everything that is decreed for the Muslim is best for him.

12. Enumerate the blessings of Allah and be thankful for them.

13. You are better off than many others.

14. Relief comes from one hour to the next.

15. In both times of hardship and ease, one should turn to supplication and prayer.

16. Calamities should strengthen your heart and reshape your outlook in a positive sense.

17. Indeed with each difficulty there is relief.

18. Do not let trifles be the cause of your destruction.

19. Indeed your Lord is Oft-Forgiving.

20. Do not be angry... Do not be angry... Do not be angry.

21. Life is bread water, and shade; so do not be perturbed by a lack of any other material thing. And in the heaven is your provision, and that which you are promised. (Quran 51:22)

22. Most evil that is supposed to happen never occurs.

23. Look at those who are afflicted and be thankful.

24. When Allah loves a people, He makes them endure trials.

25. You should constantly repeat those supplications that the Prophet (pbuh) taught us to say during times of hardship.

26. Work hard at something that is productive, and cast off idleness. 27. Don't spread rumors and don't listen to them, and if you hear a rumor inadvertently, then do not believe it.

28. Your malice and your striving to seek revenge are much more harmful to your health than they are to your antagonist.

29. The hardships that befall you atone for your sins.

Why grieve when you have the six ingredients?

The author of Ease After Difficulty mentioned the story of a wise person who was afflicted by calamity. His brothers went to him and tried to console him over his loss. He answered, 'I have put together a remedy that is composed of six ingredients.' They asked him what those ingredients were, and he answered, "The first is to have a firm trust in Allah, the Almighty. The second is resigning oneself to the inescapable fact that everything that is decreed will happen and will follow its unalterable course. The third is that patience has no substitute for the positive effect it has on the afflicted. The fourth is an unwavering belief in the implications of this phrase: 'Without showing forbearance what will I accomplish?' The fifth is to ask myself, 'Why should I be a willful party to my own destruction?' The sixth is knowing that from one hour to the next, circumstances are transformed and difficulties vanish."

Do not grieve if others inflict upon you harm or pain, nor should you grieve if you are oppressed or are the subject of envy. Shaykh al-Islam (Ibn Taymiyah) said: "The believer does not seek quarrel or revenge, nor does he find blame or fault in others."

Do not despair if you face obstacles or problems; rather, forbear and be patient.

"O' time, if you have any of that leftover, from which you bring down the worthy then let me have it."

Patience, as opposed to anxiety, bears the fruit of comfort; and the one who does not voluntarily show patience will have it forced upon him by circumstances.

Al-Mutanabbi said: "Time has showered me with trouble until the arrows on my heart have formed a cover, that now when I am struck with an arrow, The blade of it strikes into the shaft of another, Now I live without a care for troubles. Since I have not profited by caring."

Do not be distressed if someone refuses you a favor, or if you are frowned upon or if the miserly person refuses you. If, by refraining from asking others, you prevent the sweat of humiliation from pouring down your face, then a wooden hut or a tent of cloth is better for you than a spacious house and a beautiful garden, material things that will only bring you worry and disquiet.

Tribulation is similar to sickness: it must run its course before it goes away, and the one who is hasty in attempting to remove it often causes it to augment and increase. It is imperative that the one who is afflicted be patient; he must wait with hope for relief, and he must be persistent in his prayers.

The fundamentals of happiness - Verses upon which to reflect

And never give up hope of Allah's Mercy. Certainly no one despairs of Allah's Mercy, except the people who disbelieve.

(Quran 12:87) And who despairs of the Mercy of his Lord except those who are astray? (Quran 15:56)

Surely, Allah's Mercy is [ever] near unto the good-doers. (Quran 7:56) You know not, it may be that Allah will afterward bring some new thing to pass.

It may be that you dislike a thing which is good for you and that you like a thing which is bad. For you. Allah knows but you do not know. (Quran 2:216)

Allah is Who sends down the rain after they have despaired, and spreads abroad His Mercy. (Quran 42:28)

And they used to call on Us with hope and feat: and used to humble themselves before Us. (Quran 21:90)

Your best companion is a book

An activity that brings about joy is for you to read a book and develop your mind through the acquisition of knowledge.

Al-Jaahi, an Arab writer from centuries ago, advised one to repel anxiety through the reading of books: "The book is a companion that does not praise you and does not entice you to evil. It is a friend that does not bore you, and it is a neighbor that causes you no harm. It is an acquaintance that desires not to extract from you favors through flattery, and it does not deceive you with duplicity and lies. When you are poring through the pages of a book, your senses are stimulated and your intellect sharpens... Through reading the biographies of others, you gain an appreciation of common people while learning the ways of kings. It can even be said that you sometimes learn from the pages of a book in a month, that which you do not learn from the tongues of men in a century. All this benefit yet no loss in wealth and no need to stand at the door of the teacher who is waiting for his fees or to learn from someone who is lower than you in manners.

The book obeys you by night as it does by day both when you are traveling and when you are at home. A book is not impaired by sleep nor does it tire in the late hours of the night. It is the teacher who is there for you whenever you are in need of it, and it is the teacher who, if you refuse to give to it, does not refuse to give to you. If you abandon it, it does not decrease in obedience. And when all turn against you showing you enmity, it remains by your side. As long as you are remotely attached to a book it suffices you from having to keep company with those that are idle. It prevents you from sitting on your doorstep and watching those who pass by. It saves you from mixing with those that are frivolous in their character, foul in their speech, and woeful in their ignorance. If the only benefit of a book was that it keeps you from foolish daydreaming and prevents you from frivolity, it would certainly be considered a true friend who has given you a great favor."

Sayings that deal with the virtues of books

Abu 'Ubaydah said: "Al-Muhallab gave his son the following advice: 'O' son, do not linger in the marketplace unless you are visiting the maker of armor or the book vendor.'"

"Forty years have passed, and I have not dozed off in the day or in the night...except that a book was resting on my chest."

Ibn al-Jahm said: "If I feel drowsy when it is time to sleep -and wasteful is the sleep that exceeds one's needs -I take up a book from the books of wisdom and I find bliss in coming across a pearl (of wisdom). I am more alert when I am happily engaged in reading and learning than I am when I hear the braying of the donkey or the shrill noise of something breaking."

He also said: "If I find a book to be agreeable and enjoyable, and if I deem it to be beneficial you will see me hour after hour checking how many pages are left, from fear of being close to the end. And if it is many volumes with a great number of pages, my life and my happiness are complete."

And the best, highest, and worthiest of books is: [This is the] Book [the Quran] sent down unto you [O' Muhammad], so let not your breast be narrow therefrom that you warn thereby, and a reminder unto the believers. (Quran 7:2)

The benefits of reading

1. Reading repels anxiety and grief.

2. While busy reading one is prevented from delving into falsehood.

3. Habitual reading makes one too busy to keep company with the idle and the inactive.

4. By reading often, one develops eloquence and clarity in speech.

5. Reading helps to develop the mind and purify its thoughts.

6. Reading increases one in knowledge and improves both memory and understanding.

7. By reading, one benefits from the experiences of others: the wisdom of the wise and the understanding of scholars.

8. By reading often, one develops the ability to both acquire and process knowledge and to learn about the different fields of knowledge and their applications to life.

9. One's faith will increase when one reads beneficial books, especially books written by practicing Muslim writers. The book is the best giver of sermons and it has a forceful effect in guiding one towards goodness and away from evil.

10. Reading helps to relax one's mind from distraction and to save one's time from being wasted.

11. By reading often, one gains a mastery over many words and learns the different constructions of sentences; moreover, one improves his ability to grasp concepts and to understand what is written 'between the lines.'

"Nourishment of the soul is in concepts and meanings, And not in food and drink."

Pause to reflect

Umar (may Allah be pleased with him) said: "We have found that the best life is that which is accompanied by patience."

He also said: "The best life that we have experienced, is that of patience, and if patience were a man, he would be most generous."

Ali (may Allah be pleased with him) said: "Truly, patience is to faith as the head is to the body. If the head is severed the body becomes wasted."

Then, he raised his voice and said: "Verily, there is no faith in the man who has no patience."

"Patience is a treasure from the treasures of goodness, a treasure that Allah does not give away except to a slave (of

His) whom He regards as being worthy."

Umar ibn 'Abdul 'Aziz said: "Whenever Allah gives a blessing to one of His slaves and then removes it from him and supplants it with patience, then that which replaces is invariably better than that which is being replaced."

Sulayman ibn al-Qaasim said: "The reward for every deed other than patience is known."

Allah, the Exalted said: Only those who are patient shall receive their rewards in full, without reckoning. (Quran 39:10)

Do not grieve - There is another life to come

The day will come when Allah will gather together the first of the creation and the last of it. The knowledge of this occurrence alone should reassure you of Allah's justice. So whoever's money is usurped here shall find it there; whoever is oppressed here shall find justice carried out there; and whoever oppresses here shall find his punishment there. Immanuel Kant, the German philosopher, said, "The drama of this life is not complete; there must be a second scene to it, for we see the tyrant and his victims without seeing justice being executed. We see the conqueror and the subjugated without the latter finding any revenge. Therefore there must be another world where justice will be carried out."

Ash-Shaykh 'Ali at-Tantawi, commenting on this, said: "This statement suggests a confession from this foreigner (to Islam), of the existence of a Hereafter where judgment will take place."

An Arab poet said: "If the minister and his delegates rule despotically, and the judge on earth is unjust in his judgments. Then woe, followed by woe after woe upon the judge of the earth from the judge Who is above." This Day shall every person be recompensed for what he earned. No injustice [shall be done to anybody]. (Quran 40: 17)

Do not feel overly stressed when work piles up

Robert Louis Stevenson said: "Every person is capable of performing his daily tasks, no matter how difficult they are, and every person is capable of living happily during his day until the sun sets: and this is the meaning of life."

Stephen Leacock said: "The young child says: when I will become a bigger boy. The boy says: when I become a teenager, and when that time comes, he says: when I will marry. What about after marriage? And what comes after all of these stages? One's thoughts constantly follow the tune of the following: when I will be able to retire. But when one actually reaches old age and looks back, he is scorched by a cold wind. He lost out on his whole life that dwindled away without ever living inside of it. And thus we learn, only when it is too late, that life is to be lived in every breathing minute and hour."

Such is the state of those who put off repenting from their sins.

One of our pious predecessors said: "'I warn you of delaying and saying that I will do it later, for this is a phrase that prevents one from doing good and causes one to fall behind in deeds of righteousness."

Leave them to eat and enjoy, and let them be preoccupied with hope. They will come to know! (Quran 15:3)

The French philosopher, Montaigne, said: "My life was filled with bad luck that never showed mercy." I assert that despite their knowledge and intelligence many famous thinkers knew nothing of the wisdom behind their own creation. They were not guided by the teachings that Allah sent through His Messenger, Muhammad (pbuh).

And he for whom Allah has not appointed light for him there is no light. (Quran 24:40)

Verily, We showed him the way, whether he be grateful or ungrateful. (Quran 76:3)

Dante said: "Consider that this day will not occur again." Better and more beautiful and complete is the hadith: "Pray as if it is your farewell prayer."

Whoever puts it into his mind that today is his last day, will make a fresh repentance, will do good deeds, and will strive to be obedient to his Lord, the Almighty and His Messenger (pbuh).

Grieve not and ask yourself the following questions

1. Do I put off living in the present because of fears and apprehensions about the future or because of hopes of the magical garden beyond the horizon?

2. Do I embitter my present life by mulling over events that occurred in the past?

3. Do I wake up in the morning with an intention of spending my day usefully?

4. Do I find that I am benefiting from my life when I try to concentrate on a present situation or task?

5. When will I begin to live in the present moment without worrying too much about the past and future? Next week? Tomorrow? Or today?

Do not despair when you face a difficult situation

If you find yourself in a tough situation do the following:

1. Ask yourself what is the worst that can happen?

2. Prepare yourself to cope and deal with that worst-case scenario.

3. If something bad does occur, meet it with calm nerves in order to deal with the situation better.

Those [i.e. believers] unto whom the people [hypocrites] said: 'Verily, the people [pagans] have gathered against you [a great army], therefore, fear them.'

But it [only] increased them in Faith, and they said: 'Allah [Alone] is Sufficient for us, and He is the Best Disposer of affairs [for us]. (Quran 3:173)

Contemplate these verses

And whosoever fears Allah and keeps his duty to Him, He will make a way for him to get out [from every difficulty]. And He will provide him from [sources] he never could imagine. And whosoever puts his trust in Allah then He will suffice him. (Quran 65:2-3) Allah will grant after hardship, ease)   (Quran 65:7)

The Prophet (Blessings and Peace be upon him) said: "And know that victory comes with patience, and with hardship there is a way out, and with difficulty comes ease."

In another hadith the Prophet (pbuh) related that Allah said: "I am with my slave's thoughts about Me, so let him think of Me as he chooses."

Allah will suffice YOU against them. And He is the All-H eare1 the All-Knower. (Quran 2:137)

And put your trust in the Ever Living One Who dies not. (Quran 25:58)

Perhaps Allah may bring a victory or a decision according to His Will. (Quran 5:52)

None besides Allah can avert it, [or advance it, or delay it]. (Quran 53:58)

Depression weakens the body and the soul

Dr. Alexis Carlyle, a Nobel-laureate in medicine, said: "Working people who do not know how to deal with anxiety and stress are more prone than others are to a premature death." Indeed, everything that takes place occurs according to a divine decree.

A person must nonetheless take the necessary steps to avoid difficulties, and so Carlyle rightly points out that anxiety is one of the factors that lead to the body being damaged.

Depression: A cause of ulcers

"You will not be afflicted by an ulcer by virtue of what you eat, but instead by virtue of what eats you." This is a quote taken from Dr. Joseph F. Mantagno's book, The Problem of Nervousness.

The renowned Arab poet Al-Mutanabbi said: '"And stress transforms obesity into scrawniness, it whitens the hair of that young man and makes him a mess."

And according to Life magazine, ulcers rank tenth in the list of deadly diseases.

Some other effects of depression

I recently read the translation of Dr. Edward Bodowlski's book.

Stop Worrying and Seek Betterment. Here are some of the chapter titles from his book:

- What Anxiety does to the heart?

- High Blood Pressure Feeds off of Anxiety

- Anxiety may be the Cause of some Forms of Rheumatism

- As a Favor to your insides, Seek to Decrease the Level of your Anxiety

- How Anxiety can be considered a Cause of the Common Cold

- Anxiety and the Thyroid Gland

- The Victim of Diabetes and Anxiety

Dr. Carl Maninger, a specialist in psychology, wrote a book called Man Against Himself (In it, he says: "'Dr. Maninger will not give you the principles of how to avoid anxiety, but instead he will give you an astonishing report on how we destroy our own body and minds through anxiety and nervousness, malice and rancor, fear, and feelings of revenge."

And those who pardon men; Allah loves the good-doer. (Quran 3:134) Among the more salient lessons that we should learn from this verse is that we should have a sound heart, peace of mind, calm nerves, and a feeling of happiness.

The French philosopher Montaigne once said: "I wish to help you in dealing with your problems with my hands, but not with my liver and lungs."

What depression and anger do

Doctor Russell Cecil of Cornell University mentioned four widespread causes of arthritis:

1. Marital strife.

2. Financial difficulties and depression.

3. Loneliness and anxiety.

4. Malice and rancor.

Doctor William Mark Gaungil, while addressing the Federation of American Dentists, remarked: "'Unhappy feelings like anxiety and fear possibly affect the distribution of calcium in the body, and in consequence, can lead to tooth decay."

Bear your hardships with serenity

Dale Carnegie said: "African-Americans that live in the South along with the Chinese rarely fall prey to those heart diseases that result from anxiety. This can be attributed to the serene and casual way in which they lead their lives."

He also said: "The number of Americans that make suicide attempts is greater than the number of those who die as a result of the five most deadly diseases combined." This is a startling statistic that should not be taken lightly.

Hold ta good opinion of your Lord

William James said: "God forgives us our sins, but our nervous systems do not." Ibn al-Wazeer wrote in his book Al-Awaaim Al-Qawaaim: "Verily, to be hopeful of Allah's mercy opens the doors of optimism for one of His slaves, making him more avid in worship, and inspiring him to be more enthusiastic in performing voluntary acts of worship and racing to perform good deeds." This is true, especially because some people are not moved to do good deeds except when they recall Allah's mercy, forgiveness, and generosity.

As a consequence of reflecting on these qualities, they seek closeness to Allah through diligently performing good deeds.

When your thoughts wander

Thomas Edison said: "'There is no subterfuge that one may resort to in order to flee from his thoughts."

One can confirm the accuracy of this statement from experience, for even when reading or writing, one is constantly diverted by inappropriate thoughts. One of the best means of controlling such thoughts is to work at something that is at once interesting and useful.

Embrace constructive criticism

Andre Moro said: "Everything that is in harmony with our personal inclinations appears to us as a truth, and everything else only serves to provoke our anger."

A prime example of this is when we are given advice or criticism. For the most part, we adore praise and our spirits are lifted when we are the objects of such attentions, even if we are praised for the wrong reasons.

On the other hand, we hate criticism and disparagement, even if what is said about us happens to be true. And when they are called to Allah [i.e. His Words, the Quran] and His Messenger, to judge between them, lo! A party of them refuse [to come] and turn away. But (/the right is with them, they come to Him willingly with submission.   (Quran 24:48-49)

William James said: "When you make a resolute decision to do something on any given day, you will be totally rid of worries that seize and subjugate you concerning the results of your endeavors."

What he means is that when you make a judicious decision based on logic and a sound premise, then you should carry out that decision. Furthermore, you must not give way to doubts, for doubts beget nothing but more doubts. And then afterwards, do not look behind.

An Arab poet said: "If you are of sound judgment show resolution, for ill judgment is in hesitation."

Showing courage in making decisions can save you from anxiety and confusion. And when the matter is resolved on, then (if they had been true to Allah, it would have been better for them. (Quran 4 7:2 1)

Dr. Richard Cabot of Harvard University wrote in his book How Humans Live: "As a physician, I am a proponent of work as a remedy for those who suffer from nervousness that results from doubts, fears, and indecisiveness. Work inspires bravery; it was self confidence that made Emerson so superb."

Then when the [Friday congregational] prayer is finished, you may disperse through the land, and seek the Bounty of Allah [by working, etc.])   (Quran 62:10)

George Bernard Shaw said: "Perhaps the secret of depression is in allowing yourself to have time for superfluous thought, especially in whether you are happy or not. Don't allow such thoughts to creep into your mind; rather, you should remain steadfast in working. When you apply yourself to a serious task, your blood will begin to circulate and your mind will be spurred into action.

You will find that your new life has quickly been removed of anxiety and worrisome thoughts. Work, and do so on a continual basis; for this is the most inexpensive remedy available on the face of the earth and the most effective." And say [O'Muhammad] 'do deeds! Allah will see your deeds, and [so will] His Messenger and the believers. · (Quran 9:105)

A wise saying of the Arabs goes: "Life is too short to make it even shorter through disputes." He [Allah] will say: 'What number of years did you stay on earth? 'They will say: 'We stayed a day or part of a day. Ask of those who keep account.' He [Allah] will say: 'You stayed not but a little, (if you had only known.' (Quran 24:112-114)

Most rumors are baseless

General George Kruk, known for his subjugation of the native Indians, wrote the following on page 77 of his famous journal: "Almost all of the misery and anxiety of the Indians originates from their imagination and not from reality."

They think that every cry is against them. (Quran 63:4)

Had they marched out with you, they would have added to you nothing except disorder, and they would have hurried about in your midst [spreading corruption] and sowing sedition among you. (Quran 9:47)

Professor Hawks of Columbia University said, "Either there is or there isn't a remedy for a given problem. If a remedy does exist for a specific problem, find it; and if not then don't bother yourself about it."

And in an authentic hadith the Prophet (pbuh) said: "Allah has not sent down a sickness except that He has also sent down for it a cure. He knows it who knows it, and he is ignorant of it who is ignorant of it (so even if the most famous doctor is ignorant of it, it still exists)."

Gentleness averts confrontations

A Japanese teacher said to his pupils, "To bow is to be like the willow, and to not return force is to be like the oak tree."

And in a hadith the Prophet (pbuh) said: "The believer is like the green plant; the wind blows it to the left and to the right."

The wise person is like water, for water does not crash into a rock, trying to pass through it. Instead, it comes to it from the left and from the right, from above and from below. In another hadith, the Prophet (Blessings and Peace be upon him) said: "The believer is like a camel whose reins are on its nose. If it were made to kneel on a rock, it would do so."

Yesterday will never return

In order that you may not be sad over matters that you fail to get. (Quran 57:23)

Adam said to Musa (Moses) may peace be upon them, "Do you blame me for that which Allah had decreed upon me forty years before He created me."

Concerning this last saying, the Prophet (pbuh) said: "Adam overcame Musa in his arguments - Adam overcame Musa in his arguments -Adam overcame Musa in his arguments."

Search for happiness inside of you, and not around you or outside of you.

The prolific English poet, Milton said: "Verily, the mind on its own is capable of transforming paradise into hell and hell into paradise!"

Al-Mutanabbi wrote: "The one who is talented suffers because of (his unbalanced genius) while he is rich, meanwhile the ignorant one is poor, and yet he is smiling."

This life does not deserve our grief. Napoleon exclaimed in Saint Helena: "I have not known (even) six happy days in my whole life."

The Caliph, Hisham ibn 'Abdul-Malik, said: "I have attempted to recall and enumerate the number of happy days in my life, and I have found them to be thirteen in total."

And his father would often repine and say, "Would that I had never become the Caliph."

The eminent preacher Ibn Sammack once visited Haroon Ar-Rasheed. The latter felt thirsty and asked for water to drink. Ibn Sammack said, "O' Ruler of the faithful, if you were refused this drink, would you bargain for it with half of your empire?" He said, "Yes."

When he finished drinking it, Ibn Sammack followed up with another question, "If, due to some sickness, you were unable to discharge this drink (through urine), would you pay half of your empire's wealth to be able to remove it from your body?" He answered, "Yes." Ibn Sammack then said, "Therefore, there is no good in a kingdom that is not even equal to a drink of water."

The whole world and whatever is in it has no value, weight, or meaning if it is devoid of faith. Iqbal said:

"When faith is lost then so is peace, and there is no life for the one, who is not enlivened by religion, whoever is pleased with a life bereft of faith

Has made total ruin to be life's substance."

Emerson concluded his essay on self-reliance with the following: "Political triumph increase in wage, a cure to your sickness, or a return to happy days -these all seem to loom for you in the horizon.

But don't believe it all because things will not be as you expected them to be, and because nothing can bring you peace except yourself."

Come back to your Lord. Well-pleased [yourself) and well-pleasing unto Him! Enter you then, among My honored slaves. (Quran 89:28-29)

A renowned philosopher and novelist said, "The indispensability of removing wicked notions from our thoughts is more critical than that of removing tumors and diseases from our bodies."

And there are more warnings in the Quran about diseases of ideas and beliefs than there are concerning bodily ailments.

The French philosopher Montaigne said: "A person is not influenced by what happens as much as he is by his opinion regarding what happens."

And in the following hadith, the Prophet (pbuh) supplicated: "O'Allah, make me pleased with Your decree, so that I may know that whatever has befallen me was not meant to miss me, and what has passed me by, was not meant to be in my lot."

Ponder these points

Do not be sad, because sadness causes you to regret the past, to have misgivings concerning the future, and to make you waste away your present. Do not be sad, because it causes the heart to contract, the face to frown, the spirit to weaken, and hope to vanish. Do not be sad, because your sadness pleases your enemy, angers your friend, and makes the jealous rejoice. Do not be sad, because by being sad, you are complaining against the divine decree and showing vexation at what is written for you.

Do not be sad, because grief cannot return to you the one that is lost or is gone away. It cannot resurrect the dead it cannot change fate, or bring any benefit whatsoever. Do not be sad, because sadness is often from the devil and is a kind of hopelessness.

Have We not opened your breast for you [O' Muhammad]? And removed from you your burden, which weighed down on your hack? And raised high your fame? So verily, with the hardship, there is relief. So when you have finished [from your occupation], then stand up for worship [i.e. stand up for prayer]. (Quran 94:1-8)

As long as you have faith in Allah, do not be sad

Faith in Allah, the Almighty, is to happiness and peace, while disbelief is to confusion and misery. I have read about many intelligent people of a certain kind, some who might even be called geniuses, geniuses though whose hearts are bereft of the light of guidance.

James Allen, author of How Man Thinks, said: "Man will come to know that each time he changes his opinions and thoughts concerning things and other people those same things and people will in their part also change. Suppose someone to have changed his thinking, and we will be astonished to learn how quickly the state of his material life changes. Therefore the sacred thing that shapes our goals is our own selves."

Regarding incorrect thinking and its effects, Allah the Exalted, says: You thought that the Messenger and the believers would never return to their families; and that seemed fair in your hearts, and you did think an evil thought and you became a useless people going for destruction. 'Indeed the affair belongs wholly to Allah. (Quran 3:154)

James Allen also said: "Everything that a person accomplishes is a direct result of his personal thinking. And man is capable of triumphing and of achieving his goals through his thinking he will remain weak and miserable if he refuses to acknowledge this."

Do not grieve over trivialities for the entire world is trivial

A righteous person was once thrown into a lion's cage, and Allah then saved him from its claws. He was later asked, "What were you thinking about at the time."

He said, "I was considering the saliva of a lion whether it is considered by scholars to be pure or impure."

Allah described those who were with the Prophet (Blessings and Peace be upon him) according to their intentions: Among you are some that desire this world and some that desire the Hereafter. (Quran 3:152)

Ibn al-Qayyim mentioned that a person's value is measured according to his determination and his goals. A wise person once said words to the same effect:

"Inform me of a man's determination and I will tell you what kind of man he is."

A vessel capsized at sea, and a worshipper was hurled into the water. He began to make ablution, one limb at a time. He managed to get to shore and was saved. He was asked about the ablution and why he made it, to which he replied, "I wanted to make ablution so that I would die in a state of purity."

Imam Ahmad during the pangs of death, was pointing to his beard while others were making his ablution for him, reminding them not to miss a spot.

So Allah gave them the reward of this world, and the excellent reward of the Hereafter. (Quran 3:148)

Do not grieve when you are shown overt enmity, for if you forgive and forget, you will have achieved nobility in this world and honor in the next.

But whoever forgives and makes reconciliation his reward is due from Allah. (Quran 42:40)

Shakespeare said words to the effect of, "Don't light the oven too much for your enemy in order not to bum yourself by the flame."

Someone said to Saalim ibn Abdullah ibn "Umar, a scholar from the early generations of Islam, "You are an evil man." He quickly replied, "None knows me save you."

A man said in a verbal attack to Abu Bakr (may Allah be pleased with him): "By Allah, I will curse you with such curses that will enter with you into your grave." He calmly answered, "Nay, but they shall enter with you into yours."

And someone said to Amr ibn al-'Aa, "I will dedicate myself to waging war against you." 'Amr replied, "Now have you fallen into what supersedes all else, and it will be your preoccupation (i.e. your misery)."

General Eisenhower once exclaimed: "Let us not waste one minute in thought over those whom we do not love."

The mosquito said to the tree: "Remain firm, for I wish to fly away and leave you." The tree answered, "By Allah. I felt not your landing on me! Then how will I feel you when you fly away."

And when the foolish address them [with bad words] they reply back with mild words of gentleness.   (Quran 25:63) Confucius said:

"The angry man is always replete with poison."

One man asked the Prophet (Blessings and Peace be upon him) to give him advice three times. He (pbuh) answered each time: "Don't be angry."

The Prophet (pbuh) said of anger in the following hadith: "Anger is an ember from the fire."

The Devil overcomes man on three occasions: when he is angry, when he feels lust, and when he is in a state of forgetfulness.

This is how the world is

Marcus Aurelius, one of the wiser of the Roman Emperors, stated one day: "Today, I shall meet people who speak much, who are selfish, loathsome, and who love only themselves. Yet I will not be annoyed or bewildered by them, because I do not imagine the rest of the world to be any different."

Strive to help others

Aristotle said: "The ideal person is he who takes pleasure in serving others, and who is ashamed when others do things for him since showing compassion is a sign of superiority, while receiving it is a sign of failure."

More concise and to the point is the following hadith: "The Upper Hand is better than the Lower Hand."

The upper hand refers to the giving hand, and the lower one refers to the receiving hand. Do not feel deprived as long as you have a loaf of bread, a glass of water and clothes on your back a mariner once became lost at sea, and remained lost for twenty- one days. When he was saved, someone asked him what the greatest lesson was that he took away with him from the experience. He answered, "The biggest lesson that I learned from it was that if you have fresh water and sufficient food, you should never complain."

It has been said that, "Life in its entirety is a morsel of food and a drink of water. Whatever exceeds that is excess."

Jonathan Swift said that the best doctors in the world are "the proper diet doctor," "the rest doctor" and, "the doctor of happiness."

The reasoning behind Swift's comment is that corpulence is a reprehensible disease that causes the level of one's intelligence to diminish. Meanwhile, rest and moderation and happiness are satisfying forms of nourishment for the mind heart, and soul.

Blessings in disguise

Dr. Samuel Johnson said: "The habit of looking on the bright side in every circumstance is more valuable than having a large income."

See they not that they are tried once or twice every year [with different kinds of calamities, disease, famine, etc.]? Yet, they turn not in repentance, nor do they learn a lesson [from it]. (Quran 9:126)

One of our pious predecessors said to someone: "Verily, I see upon you the signs of blessings, and my advice to you is to lock your blessings up and keep them safe by being thankful."

Your Lord proclaimed: If you give thanks [by accepting Faith and worshipping none but Allah], I will give you more [of My Blessings], but if you are thankless [i.e. disbelievers], verily! My Punishment is indeed severe. (Quran 14:7)

And Allah puts forward the example of a township [Makkah], that dwelt secure and well content; its provision coming to it in abundance from every place, but it [its people] denied the Favors of Allah [with ungratefulness]. So Allah made it taste the extreme of hunger [famine] and fear, because of that [evil, i.e. denying

Prophet Muhammad] which they [its people] used to do. (Quran 16:112)

You are created unique

Dr. James Gordon Gilkee said: "The dilemma of wanting your own identity is as ancient as the beginning of history, and it is common to all human life. Similar is the problem of not wanting to be your own self, which is the source of much personal imbalance and disturbance."

Someone else said: "You are a unique entity among creation: nothing is exactly similar to you, nor are you exactly similar to anything, because the Creator has brought diversity to the creation."

Certainly, your efforts and deeds are diverse [different in aims and purposes]. (Quran 92:4)

Angelo Battero wrote thirteen books and thousands of articles related to the topic of child education.

He once wrote: "There is none more miserable than the one who grows up not being himself, who grows up imitating others in appearance and thought."

He sends down water [rain] from the sky, and the valleys flow according to their measure. (Quran 13:17)

Every person has his own idiosyncrasies talents, and abilities, so no one should fuse his personality into that of another.

Undoubtedly, you have been created with restricted means and abilities that will help you to accomplish very specific and limited goals. It has been wisely put: Read yourself and know yourself; you will then know your mission in life.

Emerson said in his essay on self-reliance: "The time will come when the knowledge of man will reach the level where his faith will be that jealousy is ignorance and imitation is suicide. And one will accept his own self, as he is, no matter what the circumstances, because that is his lot. Also, despite the fact that the world is filled with good things, one will not accomplish anything until he plants and cares for the land that was given to him. Hidden strengths that are inside of him are new to the world, and he does not know the extent of his abilities until he tries." And say [O' Muhammad]. 'Do deeds! Allah will see your deeds, and [so will] His Messenger and the believers. · (Quran 9:105) Contemplate these verses: Say: 'O' My servants, who have transgressed against themselves [by committing evil deeds and sins]! Despair not of the Mercy of Allah, verily Allah forgives all sins. Truly, He is the Most Merciful. (Quran 39:53) And those who knew they have committed Fahisha [illegal sexual intercourse etc.] or wronged themselves with evil, remember Allah and ask forgiveness for their sins; -and none can forgive sins but Allah -And do not persist in what [wrong] they have done, while they know.   (Quran 3:135)

Allah responds to the invocations of the supplicant when he calls on Me [without any mediator or intercessor]. So let them obey Me and believe in Me, so that they may be led aright. (Quran 2:186)

Allah responds to the distressed one, when he or she calls Him, and Who removes the evil, and makes you inheritors of the earth, generations after generations.

Much that in appearance is harmful is in fact a blessing

William James said: "Our handicaps help us to an extent that we never expected. If Dostoevsky and Tolstoy had not lived painful lives, they would not have been capable of writing their ageless journals. So being an orphan blind poor, or away from home and comfort are all conditions that may lead you to accomplishment and distinction, to advancement and contribution."

A poet said: "Allah can bestow His blessings through trials that are small or large, And He puts some to trial by giving them of His blessings." Even children and wealth can be the cause of misery: So let not their wealth tor their children amaze you O'Muhammad]; in reality Allah's Plan is to punish them with these things in the life of this world. (Quran 9:55)

Upon becoming crippled, Ibn Kathir was afforded the opportunity to complete his many famous books. All fifteen volumes of it, while being imprisoned at the bottom of a well. The scholars of hadith gathered hundreds and thousands of ahaadeeth (hadiths): these were people that were poor, people that were strangers to the word 'home.' A righteous person informed me that he was imprisoned for a while, and during the period of his incarceration, he memorized the entire Quran and studied forty large volumes on Islamic jurisprudence.

Abu Al-Ulaa dictated his books to others because he was blind. Many bright people, upon being removed from their positions or jobs contributed to the world in knowledge and thought much more than they ever previously did in their lives.

Francis Bacon said that, "A little philosophy makes one lean towards disbelief, and to delve into philosophy brings the mind closer to religion." And these similitudes We put forward for mankind but none will understand them except those who have knowledge [of Allah and His Signs, etc.]. (Quran 29:43)

It is only those who have knowledge among His slaves that fear Allah. (Quran 35:28)

And those who have been bestowed with knowledge and faith will say: 'Indeed you have stayed according to the Decree of Allah, until the Day of Resurrection." (Quran 30: 56)

"The true believer will never be afflicted by mental sickness." Verily, those who believe [in the Oneness of Allah and in His Messenger (Muhammad)] and work deeds of righteousness, the Most Beneficent [Allah] will bestow love for them [in the hearts of the believers]. (Quran 19:96)

Whoever works righteousness, whether male or female, while he [or she] is a true believer [of Islamic Monotheism], We shall pay them certainly a reward in proportion to the best of what they used to do [i.e. Paradise in the Hereafter]. (Quran 16:97)

And verily, Allah is the Guide of those who believe, to the straight path. (Quran 22:54)

Faith is the greatest remedy!

One of the foremost experts in psychology of our time, Dr. Carl Jung, mentioned in his book The Modern Man In Search Of Spirit: "Over the last thirty years, people from all over the world have come to me seeking advice. I treated hundreds of patient s and most of them were middle-aged or more than thirty-five years old. The problem with every one of them returned to one issue - seeking refuge in religion, and by doing so, being able to have a perspective or outlook on life. I can reasonably say that every one of them became sick because they missed out on that which religion has to offer to the believer. And the one who does not develop a true faith cannot be healed."

But whosoever turns away from My Reminder [i.e. neither believes in this Quran nor acts on its orders, etc.] verily, for him is a life of hardship. (Quran 20: 124)

We shall cast terror into the hearts of those who disbelieve, because they forgot Allah. (Quran 3:151)

In darkness, if a man stretches out his hand, he can hardly see it! And he for whom Allah has not appointed light for him, there is no light.

Do not lose hope

Allah answers the prayer of the disbeliever who is in distress; so how much more can the Muslim expect who doesn't associate partners with Him? Mahatma Gandhi, perhaps second in popularity in India only to the Buddha, was on the verge of slipping were it not for his dependence on the strength of prayer. And how do I know this? Because, he himself said, "If I didn't pray, I would have gone mad a long time ago. This was the effect of prayer, and Gandhi was not even a Muslim. Unquestionably his falsehood was great, but what kept him going was that he was on a path.

And when they embark on a ship, they invoke Allah, making their Faith pure for Him only, but when He brings them safely to land, behold, they give a share of their worship to others. (Quran 29:65)

Is not He [better than your gods] Who responds to the distressed one, when he calls Him. (Quran 27:62)

And they think that they are encircled therein, they invoke Allah, making their Faith pure for Him Alone, saying: 'If You [Allah] deliver us from this, we shall truly be of the grateful. · (Quran 10: 22)

Despite a thorough search through the biographies of Muslim scholars, Muslim historians, and Muslim writers as a group, I have failed to find a single one of them who fell prey to anxiety, confusion, and mental illnesses. The reason is that they lived in peace and serenity, and that they lived uncomplicated lives that were free from all forms of affectation.

But those who believe and do righteous good deeds, and believe in that which is sent down to Muhammad, for it is the truth from their Lord, He will expiate from them their sins, and will make good their state. (Quran 47:2)

Contemplate the following statement of Ibn Hazim: "There is only one day separating kings and me. As for yesterday, their taste of it has vanished, and both they and I equally fear what tomorrow will bring. Thus there is only today. And what will today bring?"

The Prophet (Blessings and Peace be upon him) said: "O' Allah, I ask you for goodness today: in its blessings, success, light, and guidance."

O' you who believe! Take your precautions. (Quran 4:71) And let him be careful and let no man know of you.

(Quran 18:19)

And they said nothing but: 'Our Lord, Forgive us our sins and our transgressions, establish our feet firmly, and give us victory over the disbelievers. (Quran 3:147)

Don't be sad - Life is shorter than you think

Dale Carnegie related a story of a man Who had an ulcer that became aggravated to a dangerous level. Doctors informed him that he had very little time left to live. They insinuated that it would be wise for him to make funeral arrangements. Suddenly, Hani - the patient- made a spontaneous decision: He thought to himself that if he had such little time left to live, why not enjoy it to the utmost? He thought. "How often have I wished to travel around the world before I die. This is certainly the chance to realize my dreams." He bought his ticket and when the doctors became aware of his plans, they were shocked.

They said to him. "We most strongly remonstrate with you and warn you: If you go forward on this journey you will be buried at the bottom of the ocean." Their arguments were in vain and he only answered. "No nothing of the sort will happen. I have promised my relatives that I will come back to be buried in the family plot."

He thus began his trip of mirth and joy. He wrote to his wife saying, "I eat the most delectable of dishes on the cruise ship. I read poetry, and I eat tasty fatty foods that I have hitherto refrained from. I have enjoyed life during this period more than I have in my entire previous life."

Dale Carnegie claimed that the man became cured of his sickness and that the energizing path he took is one that is successful in defeating disease and pain. The moral: happiness cheerfulness, and calmness are often more efficacious than doctors' pills.

As long as you have life's basic necessities - Don't be sad

And it is not your wealth, nor your children that bring you nearer to Us, but only he who believes [in the Islamic Monotheism] and does righteous deeds; as for such, there will be twofold reward for what they did, and they will reside in the high dwellings [Paradise] in peace and security. (Quran 34:37)

Dale Carnegie said: "Statistics have proven that stress and anxiety are the number one killer s in America. As a result of the last world war, one third of a million of our soldiers were killed. In the same period heart disease was the cause of two million deaths. And from this latter group, stress, anxiety, and nervous tension were the source of sickness for one million people."

Yes, heart disease is one of the main reasons that prompted Dr. Alexis Carlyle to say: "Working people who do not know how to deal with stress die prematurely.'

Though the reasoning and logic that prompted Carlyle to say this are sound, we must still remember: And no person can ever die except by Allah's Leave and at an appointed time. (Quran 3:145)

Asians rarely fall prey to diseases of the heart. They are people who live life with tranquility and calmness. On the other hand, you will find that the number of doctors who die of heart attacks is twenty times more than the number of farmers who die of the same cause. Doctors live a tough and stress filled life, for which they pay a heavy price.

Contentment repels sadness

The Messenger of Allah (Blessings and Peace be upon him) said: "We do not say other than that which pleases our Lord."

Upon you is a sacred duty to surrender yourself to what is preordained for you. If you fulfill this duty, you will be successful in the long run.

Your only escape is to believe in preordainment, since whatever has been decreed must inevitably take place. No subterfuge or artifice can protect you from it.

Emerson said: "From where has the idea come to us which says that a luxurious stable life, free from obstacles and hardships, creates prosperous and great men? The case is quite the opposite. Those who have made a habit of living the easy life will continue to further develop lazy habits as they go on in life. History witnesses that greatness has surrendered its reins to men of different backgrounds. From these backgrounds are environments that have both good and bad, or environments where good and bad cannot be distinguished. And from such environments have sprouted up men who have carried great responsibilities on their shoulders without ever negligently casting them off."

Who were those that carried the flag of Divine guidance in the early days of Islam? They were the freed slaves, the poor, and the destitute. And most of the people who stood defiantly against them were the nobles, the chiefs, and the rich.

And when Our Clear Verses are recited to them, those who disbelieve [the rich and strong among the pagans of Quraysh who lived a life of luxury say to those who believe [the weak, poor Companions of Prophet Muhammad]: 'which of the two groups [i.e. believers and disbelievers] is best in position and station. (Quran 19:73) and they say: 'We are more in wealth and in children, and we are not going to be punished. (Quran 34:35)

Thus We have tried some of them with others that they might say: 'is it these [poor believers] that Allah has favored from amongst us?' Does not Allah know best those who are grateful? (Quran 6:53)

And those who disbelieve [strong and wealthy] say of those who believe [weak and poor]: 'had it [Islamic Monotheism to which Muhammad is inviting mankind] been a good thing. (Quran 46:11)

Those who were arrogant said: "Verily, we disbelieve in that which you believe in. The Quran would have been instead sent down to some great man in our town." I often recall the verses of Antara, in which he establishes that his worth is in his character and deeds, and not in his lineage or connections. He said: "Despite being a slave, I am a noble chief; and despite being black in color, I have a white character." If you lose a limb, you still have others to compensate for it.

Ibn Abbaas (may Allah be pleased with him) said: "If Allah removes the light from my eyes, My tongue and ears still have in them light. My heart is intelligent and my mind is not crooked, and my tongue is sharp like a warrior's sword."

When harm befalls you, perhaps there is a benefit that comes with it, a benefit that you cannot perceive. And it may be that you dislike a thing which is good for you. (Quran 2:216)

Bashhar ibn Burd said: "My enemies disparage me, and the defect is in them, it is not a disgrace to be called defective. If a person can see gallantry and truth, Blindness in the eyes will not be a hindrance.

In blindness I see rewards savings, and protection, and for these three, I am most needy."

Observe the difference between what Ibn 'Abbaas or Bashhar said and what Ibn Abdul Quddoos said when he became blind: "Farewell to the world; the old man Who is blind Has no share whatsoever of this life. He dies and people consider him to be of the living, false hopes have betrayed him from the beginning."

All Divine decrees will come to pass, both upon the one who accepts them and upon the one who rejects them. The difference is that the former wil find reward and happiness while the latter will find only sin and misery.

'Umar ibn 'Abdul-'Aziz wrote to Maymoon ibn Mehran: "You have written to console me for losing 'Abdul-Malik. For this matter I had been in waiting, and when it finally came to pass, I had no misgivings about it."

The days rotate in bringing good and bad. It has been related that Imam Ahmad visited Baqi ibn Mukhalid while he was sick and said to him: "O' Baqi, rejoice in Allah's reward. The days of health are devoid of sickness and the days of sickness are devoid of health."

This means that during days of health one never contemplates sickness, for plans and ambitions then increase, as do hopes and desires.

During days of severe sickness, however, one forgets matters that pertain to times of health; weak despair encamps itself within the sick soul, and thus hopelessness prevails. Allah, the Exalted, said: "if We give man a taste of Mercy from Us, and then withdraw it from him, verily! He is despairing, ungrateful. (Quran 11:9-11)

Commenting on this verse, Ibn Kathir wrote: "Allah is describing man and the base characteristic that he is the possessor of (with the exception of those believers upon whom Allah has bestowed His mercy). In general if man is afflicted with hardship after ease, he becomes hopeless of ever seeing good in the future; he shows disdain for the past- as if he never experienced good days -and despair for the future as if he never expected succor and relief."

Travel throughout Allah's wide earth

It has rightly been said that traveling drives away worries. Ramhumuzi enumerated in his book. The Noble Scholar of Hadeeth, the various benefits of traveling for the purpose of seeking knowledge. He was refuting those who think that no tangible benefit can be derived by traveling through the lands. He said: "There is much profit to be derived from seeing new lands and new houses, in seeing beautiful gardens and fields, in seeing different faces and coming across different languages and colors, and in witnessing the wonders of different countries. The peace that one finds under the shades of large trees is unparalleled. Eating in the mosques, drinking from streams, and sleeping wherever one finds a place when night comes - these all instill affability and humbleness in a person. The traveler befriends all those whom he loves for Allah's sake and he has no reason to flatter or to be artificial. Add to these benefits all of the happiness that the traveler's heart feels when he reaches his destination, and the thrill he experiences after having overcome all of the obstacles that were on his way. If those who are averse to leaving their homelands knew all of this, they would learn that all of the individual pleasures of the world are combined in the noble pursuit of traveling. There is nothing more enjoyable to a traveler than the beautiful sights and the wonderful activities that are part of traveling through Allah's wide earth. And the non-traveler is deprived of all of this."

Contemplate these Prophetic sayings

"If Allah loves a people, He tests them. Whoever is pleased, for him there is pleasure, and whoever is angry, upon him there is wrath."

"The most harshly tested people are the Prophets followed in succession by those who are best after them. A man is tested according to his religion. If his religion is strong with him, his test will be more intense. If his religion is weak with him, he will be tested according to the level of his religion. (Allah's) slave will continually be tested until he is left to walk on the earth without a mistake (to have to account for)."

"Wonderful is the situation of the believer. All of his affairs are good (for him)! And this is only for the believer. If good befalls him, he is thankful, and that is good for him. If harm afflicts him, he is patient, and that is good for him."

"And know that if the entire Nation were to gather upon benefiting you with something, they would only benefit you with something that Allah has (already) written for you.

And if they were to gather upon harming you with something, they would only harm you with something that Allah has (already) written for you."

"The righteous ones are tested: first, the best of them, then the next, and so on." "The believer is like a tiny branch, the wind blows it to the right and to the left."

In the last moments of life

Abu Al-Bayrooni was a prolific thinker and writer whose pen rarely left his hand. He lived to the ripe age of seventy-eight and throughout his life he never unnecessarily took a break from reading, writing, or teaching.

A man said: "I visited Abu Al-Bayrooni when he was on his deathbed. Upon entering, I immediately recognized that he was on the verge of leaving this life.

While in that state, he said to me that there was an issue in (Islamic) inheritance law that we had discussed the last time we met and that I had said something then that he now realized was a mistake. I felt compassion for him, and asked him if it was proper for him to discuss something like that, with him being so ill. He answered. 'I know that I am leaving this world, but don't you think it is better for me to understand the issue in question than to be ignorant of it?' I then repeated to him the issue, and he started to explain it to me. After we finished our conversation, I left, and upon exiting, I heard a scream and I knew that he had died. It is only lofty souls like his that remain strong right until the end."

When Umar was bleeding to death after being stabbed, he asked his companions whether he had completed the prayer.

Ibrahim ibn al-Jarrah said: "Abu Yusuf became sick and was vacillating between wakefulness and unconsciousness. When he regained consciousness, he asked me about a religious issue. When he saw the wonder with which I received his question, he said to me, 'No matter, we will study this issue in the hope that the knowledge of it perpetuates until it becomes the cause of saving someone.'"

This is how our pious predecessors were. Every time they revived while yet being on their deathbeds, they would talk about Islamic knowledge. Either as a teacher or as a student. How precious was knowledge to their hearts! In the last moments of their lives, they remembered neither family nor wealth; they only remembered the knowledge that was the toil of their lives. May Allah have mercy upon them! Ameen!

Do not let calamity shake you

Ahmad ibn Yusuf wrote that man positively knows that ease comes after difficulty just as the light of day comes after the dark of night. In spite of this knowledge the weaker part of his nature takes over when calamity strikes. A person who goes through trials should take steps to remedy his situation or else hopelessness takes control of him. Contemplating the patience of those who were tested in the past is a means of strengthening one's determination. He mentioned later that hardship before comfort is analogous to hunger before food: food comes at a time when it has its greatest effect on the taste buds.

Plato said: "Hardship is as beneficial to the soul as it is unwelcome in one's life. Comfort is as harmful to the soul as it is welcome in life."

When someone begins to understand his purpose in life, he will know that he is being tested either to gain reward from Allah or to gain atonement for his sins.

After reading a book written by At-Tanooki, I derived three conclusions:

1. Relief comes after hardship. This is a consistent pattern in the life of man, as consistent as the coming of morning after darkness.

2. Hardship is more beneficial to the soul of man than are comfort and ease.

3. The One who brings good and drives away evil is Allah. Know that whatever happens to you was decreed for you, and whatever you have missed out was never meant for you.

Do not grieve - This world is not worth your grief

The Prophet (Blessings and Peace be upon him) said: "If this world were worth the wing of a mosquito to Allah, He would not have given the disbeliever (even) a drink of water."

This world is not even worth the wing of a mosquito! If this is the worth of this world, why do we grieve over it?

Do not be sad: Remember that you believe in Allah

Allah has conferred a favor upon you, that He has guided you to the Faith. (Quran 49:17) One particular blessing overlooked by most people is the vantage point afforded to the believer when he is observing the disbeliever. The believer remembers Allah's favor of guiding him to Islam. He is thankful that Allah has not decreed for him to be like the disbeliever, who rebels, denies His signs, disbelieves in His perfect attributes, in His messengers, and in the Hereafter.

Furthermore, the believer performs all obligatory acts of worship. Per aps his execution of those acts is not perfect, yet simply performing them is in itself a great blessing. It is a blessing for which few are grateful.

Is then he who is a believer like him who is Faasiq [disbeliever and disobedient to Allah]? Not equal are they! (Quran 32:18) Some commentators of the Quran have said that among the pleasures of Paradise for the believers is to be able to look upon the people of the Fire and then thank their Lord for what He has given them.

Pause to reflect

There is none worth of worship except Allah. This means that none truly deserves, or has the right to be worshipped, except Allah, the Almighty, All-High, since He alone possesses those perfect qualities that are associated with omnipotence, divinity, and godhood.

The spirit and secret of this monotheistic phrase is to single out. Our love is pure for none except Him, and everyone other than Him is only loved as a by-product of our love for Him, or as a means of increasing our love for Him.

Therefore we must fear Allah Alone, and we must depend upon Him Alone in Him Alone do we place our hopes; and of Him Alone are we in awe. We take an oath by His name only; we repent to Him Alone; and all obedience is for Him. In times of hardship, we may invoke none but Him and we may seek refuge in none save in Him. Also, we prostrate to Him only, and when we slaughter an animal, we do it, mentioning His name only. All of the above can be summarized in one phrase: None has the right to be worshipped except Allah. This phrase is comprehensive of all forms of worship.

Despair not - Handicaps do not prevent success

An interview was published in the Arabic daily with a blind. He studied books of Arabic literature through the eyes of others. He would listen as others read to him books of history and commentaries on the classics. He used to have one of his friends read to him until 3 o'clock in the morning. Today, he is considered to be a reference book in literature and history.

A columnist wrote: "Be patient with oppressors and wrongdoers for only five minutes. After a short time, the whip will fall, the shackles will break, the prisoner will be released, and the clouds will dissipate; upon you then, is only to be patient and to wait."

An Arab poet wrote: "How many calamities cause one to lose patience? But from them, the exit is with Allah.., I once met with the Mufti of Albania in Riyadh. He told me of how the ruling communists imprisoned him with hard labor for twenty years. While serving his sentence in prison, he was constantly subjected to torture, darkness, and hunger. He would secretly perform the five daily prayers in a comer of the washroom for fear of being caught. Through all of this he was patient and anticipated his reward with Allah until finally relief came. So they returned with Grace and Bounty from Allah. (Quran 3:174) Consider Nelson Mandela, the one-time President of South Africa, who for twenty-seventy years endured imprisonment. He sought freedom for his people and he struggled to break off the shackles of tyranny and oppression. He was steadfast and firm, and he almost appeared to be seeking out death.

As a result, he reached his goal and achieved his worldly glory. Allah, the Exalted, said: To them We shall pay in full [the wages of] their deeds therein. (Quran 11:15)

If you are suffering [hardships] then surely, they [too] are suffering [hardships] as you are suffering, but you have a hope from Allah [for the reward, i.e. Paradise] that for which they hope not. (Quran 4:104)

If a wound [and death] has touched you, be sure a similar wound [and death] has touched the others. (Quran 3:140)

If you embrace Islam, there is no reason for you to be sad

Miserable are those souls that are ignorant of Islam or that know Islam but have not been guided to it. Today, Muslims need a slogan or advertisement to be broadcast worldwide, for Islam is a great message that must be conveyed to the masses. The words of this slogan need to be clear, concise, and inviting because the happiness of humanity as a whole lies in this true Religion.

And whoever seek a religion other than Islam, it will never be accepted of him. (Quran 3:85)

A famous caller to Islam settled in Munich, Germany some years ago. Upon reaching the entrance of this city, he noticed a large placard. Upon it was written, "You don't know Yokohama Tires." He later put up a sign beside it and it was just as large. He wrote on it, "You don't know Islam. If you wish to know about it, call us at this number."

There was an inundation of calls from native Germans. In one year alone, thousands of people accepted Islam at this man's hands. He also established a mosque, an Islamic center, and a school.

Most human beings are confused and are in dire need of this great religion. They need Islam so that a peaceful and serene life can take the place of the chaotic one that they are presently leading. Wherewith Allah guides all those who seek His Good Pleasure to ways of peace, and He brings them out of darkness by His Will unto light and guides them to a Straight Way [Islamic Monotheism]. (Quran 5:16)

A worshipper who was found living in a remote area, and who never had prior contact with other men, said: "I never thought that anyone in the world worshipped other than Allah."

But few of My slaves are grateful. (Quran 34:13) And if you obey most of those on earth, they will mislead you far away from Allah's path. (Quran 6:116) And most of mankind will not believe even (you desire it eagerly). (Quran 12:103)

One scholar informed me that during the time when Sudan was a colony under the British Empire, a desert nomad came to the capital city, Khartoum. When he saw a British policeman walking in the center of the city, he asked a passerby, "Who is that?" He was told that the man was a foreign policeman and that he was a disbeliever. The nomad asked, "A disbeliever in what?" "A disbeliever in Allah." was the reply. Living in the desert for so long, this man's inborn nature - unspoiled by evil ideas -had remained intact, and so, when he heard something so absurd, it made him astonished and sick. He said, "And does anyone disbelieve in Allah!"

What is the matter with them that they believe not? (Quran 84:20) Then, by the Lord of the heaven and the earth, it is the truth [i.e. what has been promised to you], just as it is the truth that you can speak. (Quran 51:23)

One should think well of his Lord and should seek His favor and mercy. In an authentic hadith the Prophet (pbuh) said that our Lord laughs. After hearing this, a desert Bedouin said, "We are not bereft of a Lord who laughs well."

And He it is Who sends down the rain after they have despaired. (Quran 42:28)

Surely, Allah's Mercy is [ever] near unto the good-doers. (Quran 7:56) Yes! Certainly, the Help of Allah is near! (Quran 2:214)

By reading the biographies of successful people, one finds that they have certain things in common, whether it is in their background, their qualities, or the circumstances that surrounded their success. Here are some of the conclusions I arrived at after having read some of their biographies.

1. A person's value is based on the good he does. This is a saying of 'Ali (may Allah be pleased with him), and it means that a person's knowledge, character worship, and generosity are the yardsticks by which we measure his worth.

And verily, a believing slave is better than a [free] Mushrik [idolater], even though he pleases you. (Quran 2:221).

One's status for this life and for the Hereafter depends on his determination striving, and sacrifice.

And strive hard in Allah's Cause as you ought to strive. (Quran 22:78)

3. Every person is the maker of his own history. He writes his life's story with his good and bad deeds.

4. Life is short and passes quickly. Do not make it shorter by sinning, by worrying, or by quarrelling.

Things that bring about happiness

1. Good deeds: Whoever works righteousness, whether male or female, while he [or she] is a true believer [of Islamic Monotheism] verily, to him We will give a good life [in this world with respect, contentment and lawful provision]. (Quran 16:97)

2. A pious wife: Our Lord! Bestow on us from our wives and our offspring who will be the comfort of our eyes. (Quran 25:74)

3. A spacious house: The Prophet (Blessings and Peace be upon him) said: "O' Allah make my house spacious for me."

4. Sustenance that is derived and earned through honest mean s: The Messenger of Allah (pbuh) said: "Verily, Allah is good and pure, and He does not accept other than what is good and pure."

5. Good manners and a spirit of fellowship with people.

6. Being debt-free and not being a profligate spender.

The ingredients of happiness

1. A thankful heart and a tongue that is moist with the remembrance of Allah.

An Arab poet said: "Thankfulness remembrance, and patience, in them are blessings and rewards."

2. Another ingredient of happiness is the keeping of secrets, especially one's own secrets. Among the Arabs there is a famous story of a Bedouin who was entrusted with a secret for a fee of twenty dinars.

At first he remained true to the deal and then suddenly, in a fit of impatience, he went and returned the money - he wanted to unburden himself from the load of the secret. This is basically because secrecy requires steadfastness, patience, and willpower.

'O' my son! Relate not your vision to your brothers. · (Quran 12:5)

A bad thing is a person that he constantly feels the urge to reveal the details of his personal affairs to others. This sickness is an old one in the annals of history. The soul loves to spread secrets and disseminate stories.

You will not die before your appointed time

When their term is reached (death time), neither can they delay it nor can they advance it an hour [or a moment]. (Quran 7:34)

This verse contains within it a consolation for cowards, those that die many deaths before their actual death. This verse tells us that for every person there is an appointed time to die: it cannot be brought forward, nor can it be held back even if all of the creation were to join together in the attempt. Whoever places his hopes or trust in something or someone other than Allah, then Allah will abandon him and make that thing or person the cause of his ruin. Whoever seeks honor with Allah and does righteous deeds, Allah will honor him and bestow upon him ranking even if he has no wealth, status, or noble lineage.

In an authentic hadith, the Prophet (Blessings and Peace be upon him) advised us to repeat this phrase often: "O'Allah who is full of Majesty and Honor."

He (pbuh) also advised us to say: "O' Ever Living, O' One Who sustains and protects all that exists."

Therefore, for one's own well-being, one should invoke Allah and seek His help with these phrases, and the answer will surely then follow. In the life of a Muslim, there are three truly joyful days:

1. The day that he abjures sinning and performs his obligatory prayers in congregation.

2. The day that he repents from a sin, forsakes it, and returns to his Lord.

3. The day that he dies to meet his Lord, having performed a final deed that is both good and pure. Whosoever loves to meet Allah, Allah loves to meet them.

After having studied the life of the Prophet's Companions (may Allah be pleased with them all), I found in them five characteristics that distinguish them from others:

1. They led simple lives that were free from ostentation and extravagance.

2. Their knowledge of religious matters was as blessed as it was profound.

And more importantly, they accompanied that knowledge with practical application. It is only those who have knowledge among His slaves that fear Allah. (Quran 35:28)

3. They gave precedence to deeds of the heart over deeds that others could see. Thus, they had sincerity; they depended upon Allah; they loved Him; they hoped from Him only; and they feared none save Him. Furthermore they assiduously performed voluntary acts of worship, such as prayer and fasting. He knew what was in their hearts... (Quran 48:18)

4. They did not seek the world and its pleasures. They turned their backs in disdain on material possessions, and they reaped the fruits of this noble stance: happiness, peace of mind, and sincerity.

5. Jihad was a priority for them over other good deeds until it became a banner by which they were recognized.

And through Jihad, they annihilated their worries and troubles, because all of the following are a part of Jihad: remembrance striving, effort, and activity.

As for those who strive hard in Us [Our Cause], We will surely guide them to Our Paths. And verily, Allah is with the good doers. (Quran 29:69) In the Quran, truths and realities that are constant and do not change are mentioned concerning this life. Here are the ones that are related to the subject matter of this book. Whoever works for Allah, He will help him: If you help [in the cause of) Allah, He will help you, and make your foothold firm. (Quran 47:7)

Whoever asks of Allah, He will answer him. When one asks Allah for forgiveness. He will forgive him. Whoever places his trust in Allah, He will be sufficient for him: And whosoever puts his trust in Allah then He will suffice him. (Quran 65:3)

There are three kinds of people whose punishment is certain: those who are rebellious against Allah those who break their pledges, and those who plot evil deeds.

Then whosoever breaks his pledge, breaks only to his own harm. (Quran 48:10)

But the evil plot encompasses only him who makes it. (Quran 35:43)

Oppressors will not escape from Allah's punishment: These are their houses in utter ruin, for they did wrong. (Quran 27:52)

The fruits of righteousness are harvested both in the short and long term: So Allah gave them the reward of this world, and the excellent reward of the Hereafter. (Quran 3:148)

Whoever obeys Allah, He will love him and provide sustenance for him: Verily, Allah is the All-Provider. (Quran 51:58)

Allah will punish the enemies of his obedient slaves: Verily, We will exact retribution. (Quran 44:16)

Even in matters of religion, one finds that in spite of the negligence we are all guilty of, some of us are better than others in performing the obligatory congregational prayers regularly, in reading the Quran, in remembering Allah, and so on. These are all favors for which we should be thankful.

Adh-Dhahabi mentioned that the great scholar of hadith, Ibn Abdul Baqi, observed the people as they were leaving the central Mosque of Baghdad. He was looking for someone who in all respects he wished to change places with in life, yet he reported that he found no one: And We have preferred them above many of those whom We have created with a marked preference. (Quran 17:70)

Pause to reflect

The Messenger of Allah (pbuh) said: "Shall I not teach you words that you should say when in distress: "Allah, Allah, My Lord; I do not associate any partners with Him."

In another hadith, the Prophet (pbuh) informed us that when one is afflicted with sickness or hardship he will find relief if he says: "Allah, My Lord; He has no partner."

At times, one becomes afflicted with a severe trial. If he turns to his Lord and surrenders his will to Him without associating any partners with Him his hardship will go away.

Steps to take if you are fearful of a jealous person

Recite the last two chapters of the Quran, remember Allah, and supplicate to Him: And from the evil of the envier when he envies.

Hide or keep secret your affairs from the jealous person: "O' my sons I Do not enter by one door, but enter by different gates." (Quran 12:67)

Good manners

Be generous to a person who attempts to harm you, for perhaps he will then desist: Repel evil with that which is better. (Quran 23:96)

Good manners lead to prosperity, while bad ones lead to misery. In a hadith, the Prophet (pbuh) said: "Through good manners, one reaches the status of the person who not only fasts, but who also stands late in the night to pray."

He (pbuh) also said: "Shall I not inform you of the most beloved to me and the one seated closest to me on the Day of Resurrection: "Those of you who are best in manners."

The Prophet's (pbuh) character was the Quran. His manners were perfect.

Sleepless nights

If you toss and turn during the night without being able to fall asleep, do the following:

1. Remember Allah with Prophetic supplications or supplications taken from the Quran: Verily, in the remembrance of Allah do hearts find rest. (Quran 13:28)

2. Avoid sleeping during the day, except when you have no other choice: And have made the day for livelihood. (Quran 78:11)

3. Read or write until sleep comes: And say: 'My Lord! Increase me in knowledge. (Quran 20: 114)

4. Work hard during the day: And [it is He Who] makes the day Nushur [i.e. getting up and going about here and therefore daily work, etc., after ones sleep at night or like resurrection after ones death. (Quran 25:47)

5. Consume stimulants such as coffee and tea in moderation.

The evil consequences of sinning

Listed below are some of the evil consequences of sinning.

1. A barrier develops between Allah and the evildoer: Nay! Surely, they [evildoers] will be veiled from seeing their Lord that day. (Quran 83:15)

2. When a person perpetrates evil deeds on a continual basis, he will become despondent, losing hope of being saved.

3. The evildoer often falls into a state of depression and anxiety: The building which they built will never cease to be a cause of hypocrisy and doubt in their hearts. (Quran 9:110)

4. Fear permeates the heart of the evildoer: We shall cast terror into the hearts of those who disbelieve, because they joined others in worship with Allah. (Quran 3:151)

5. Life becomes wretched for the evildoer: verily, for him is a life of hardship. (Quran 20: 124)

6. The heart of the evildoer blackens and becomes hard: and mad e their hearts grow hard. (Quran 5:13)

7. An evildoer's face loses its light and becomes morbid: As for those whose faces will become burnt [to them will be said]: Did you reject Faith. (Quran 3:106)

8. People feel contempt for an evildoer.

9. The worldly circumstances of an evildoer become straitened: and if only they had acted according to the Torah, the Injeel [Gospel], and what has [now] been sent down to them from their Lord [the Quran], they would surely have gotten provision from above them and from underneath their feet. (Quran 5:66)

10. The wrath of Allah, a decrease in faith, and calamity -all of these are the lot of the evildoer: So they have drawn on themselves wrath upon wrath. (2:90)

But on their hearts is the Raan [covering of sins and evil deeds] which they used to earn. (Quran 83:14)

Strive for your sustenance, but don't be covetous

The Lord of the world provides for the worm in the ground: There is not a moving [living] creature on earth, nor a bird that flies with its two wings, but are communities like you. (Quran 6:38) Allah provides for the birds in the sky and for the fish in the sea: And it is He Who feeds but is not fed. (Quran 6:14)

You are worthier than a worm, bird, or fish, so do not worry about sustenance. I have known people who were stricken by poverty simply because of their distance from Allah. Some of them were rich and healthy, but instead of being thankful they turned away from obedience to Allah, they abandoned prayer, and they perpetrated major sins.

Allah took away from them their health and their wealth, replacing these with poverty, sickness, and anxiety. They were then afflicted with hardship upon hardship calamity upon calamity.

The secret of guidance

Contentment and happiness are blessings that are given only to those who follow the straight path. Muhammad (pbuh) left us upon one end of this path, and at the other end of it are the gardens of Paradise. By happiness We mean this: when one adheres to the straight path, though he may be afflicted with hardships along the way, he is confident of a happy ending and a future abode in Paradise. As a result, he will follow the Prophet (pbuh), who spoke not from his own desires, who was im1nune to the whisperings of the Devil, and whose sayings are a proof upon mankind.

For each [person], there are angels in succession before and behind him. They guard him by the Command of Allah. (Quran 13:11)

One can sense the joy of a righteous person by his mannerisms and by his treading the straight path. He knows that he has a Lord and that he has a role model in the Messenger (pbuh); he has the Book of Allah in his hand illumination in his heart, and a conscience that prompts him to do well. He is advancing to a greater state of bliss and is always striving for betterment. This is the Guidance (Allah with which he guides whosoever He will of His slaves). (Quran 6:88)

There are two paths: one that is figurative and the other that has a physical reality. The first path is that of faith, which one treads in this transient life, a life that is fraught with temptation s and desires. The second path is in the Hereafter.

Every person will have to go across that second path in order to reach Paradise. Anyone who fails will plunge into the Fire. This path or bridge is teeming with spikes. Whoever is guided to the path of faith and belief in this life will safely cross the path of the Hereafter -the speed at which he crosses will be proportional to the level of his faith. And know that if one is blessed with being guided to the straight path, his worries and anxieties will quickly vanish.

Ten gems for ta good and noble life

1. Wake up in the last third of the night to beg forgiveness from Allah: And those who pray and beg Allah's Pardon in the last hours of the night. (Quran 3:17)

2. At least once in a while, seclude yourself from people in order to contemplate.

And [those who] think deep about the creation of the heavens and the earth. (Quran 3:191)

3. Stay in the company of the righteous. And keep yourself patiently with those who call on their Lord. (Quran 18:28)

4. Remember Allah often. Remember Allah with much remembrance. (Quran 33:41)

5. Pray two units of prayer with sincerity and devotion. Those who offer their prayer with all solemnity and full submissiveness. (Quran 23:2)

6. Recite the Quran with understanding and reflection. Do they not then consider the Quran carefully? (Quran 4:82)

7. Fast on a hot dry day. He abandons his food, drink, and desire all for Me.

8. Give charity secretly. Until the left hand doesn't know what the right hand has spent.

9. Provide relief and aid to the afflicted and help and feed the animals. Whoever gives relief to a person from one of the vicissitudes of this life, Allah will relieve him from a calamity that is from the calamities of the Day of Judgment.

10. Try to be as abstemious and abstinent as possible in this fleeting world. The Hereafter is better and more lasting. (Quran 87:17) Among the delusions of Prophet Noah's son was his saying: I will betake myself to a mountain, it will save me from the water. (Quran 11:43)

If he had prayed to Allah, his outcome would have been different. And the cause of misery for An-Namrood was his saying: "I bring about life and I cause death." He tried wearing a garb that was not his and he claimed to have a quality that he did not in fact have, and thus his downfall became complete.

The key to our happiness can be summed up in one simple yet profound phrase, the Phrase of Taweed (Islamic Monotheism):

"There is none worthy of worship except Allah and Muhammad is His Messenger."

When one pronounces this phrase on earth, it will be said to him in the heavens, "You have spoken the truth."

And he [Muhammad] who has brought the truth [this Quran and Islamic Monotheism] and [those who] believed therein. (Quran 39:33) And when one lives his life in harmony with this phrase on a practical level, he will be saved from destruction shame, and the Hellfire.

And Allah will deliver those who are the pious to their places of success [Paradise]. (Quran 39:61) When one not only applies the Phrase of Taweed, but also calls others to it, his name will be remembered and he will be made victorious: And that Our hosts, they verily would be the victors. (Quran 37:173)

When one loves the Phrase of Taweed, he will be elevated in ranking and endowed with honor. But honor, power and glory belong to Allah, His Messenger, and to the believers. (Quran 63:8)

Bilal (may Allah be pleased with him) called out with the Phrase of Taweed and his situation underwent a dramatic inward change that ran parallel to his outward change of being freed from slavery. He brings them out from darkness into light. (Quran 2:257) Abu Lahab balked at and desisted from saying the Phrase of Taweed. He died in a weak and pathetic state. And whosoever Allah disgraces, none can honor him. (Quran 22:18)

The Phrase of Tawheed is an elixir that transforms the base human being into a paragon of pureness and devotion. But We have made it [this Quran] a light wherewith We guide whosoever of Our slaves We will. (Quran 42:52)

Whatever you do, do not exult in wealth acquired if you have turned your back on the Hereafter. If you do turn your back on the Hereafter, a harsh punishment and severe chastisement will lie in wait for you: "My wealth has not availed me. My power and arguments [to defend myself] have gone from me." (Quran 69:28-29) Verily, your Lord is Ever Watchful [over them]. (Quran 89:14)

Also, do not exult excessively in your child if you have forgotten your Lord. Turning away from Him is the ultimate failure. And they were covered with humiliation and misery. (Quran 2:61)

And finally, do not be complacent about your wealth if your deeds are evil, for such deeds will be your disgrace in the Hereafter. But surely the torment of the Hereafter will be more disgracing. (Quran 41:16)

And it is not your wealth, nor your children that bring you nearer to Us [i.e. pleases Allah], but only he [will please Us] who believes [in the Islamic Monotheism], and does righteous deeds. (Quran 34:37)

Say, "Who rescues you from the darknesses of the land and sea [when] you call upon Him imploring [aloud] and privately, 'If He should save us from this [crisis], we will surely be among the thankful.' "(Quran 6:63)

Say, "It is Allah who saves you from it and from every distress; then you [still] associate others with Him.

(Quran 6:64)

www.ingramcontent.com/pod-product-compliance
Lightning Source LLC
Chambersburg PA
CBHW071216080526
44587CB00013BA/1400